Bed Rest Mom

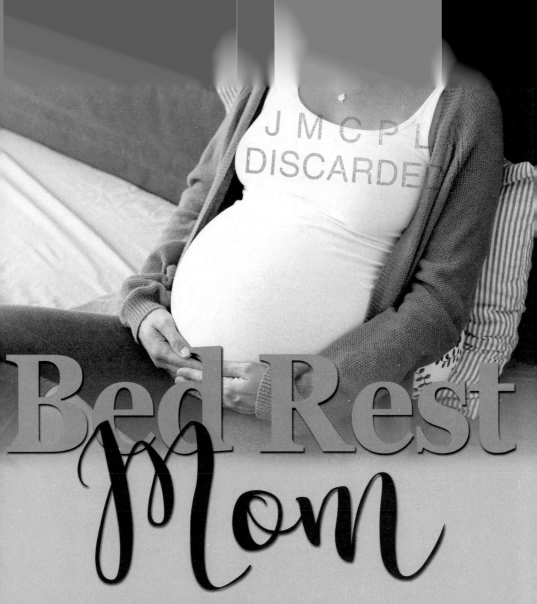

Bed Rest Mom

Surviving Pregnancy-Related Bed Rest with Your Sanity and Dignity Intact

Cynthia Lockrey

Self-Counsel Press
(a division of)
International Self-Counsel Press Ltd.
Canada   USA

Self-Counsel Press acknowledges the financial support of the Government of Canada for our publishing activities. Canadä

Printed in Canada.

First edition: 2018

Library and Archives Canada Cataloguing in Publication

Lockrey, Cynthia, author
    Bed rest mom : surviving pregnancy-related bed rest with your sanity and dignity intact / Cynthia Lockrey.

(Healthcare series)
Issued in print and electronic formats.
ISBN 978-1-77040-301-7 (softcover).—ISBN 978-1-77040-490-8 (EPUB).—ISBN 978-1-77040-491-5 (Kindle)

    1. Bed rest—Psychological aspects. 2. Pregnancy—Complications—Prevention. 3. Adjustment (Psychology). I. Title. II. Series: Self-counsel healthcare series

RG572.L63 2018   618.2'4   C2017-907600-0
                                             C2017-907601-9

Self-Counsel Press
(a division of)
International Self-Counsel Press Ltd.

Bellingham, WA   North Vancouver, BC
USA   Canada

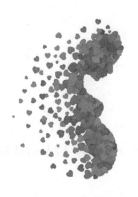

Contents

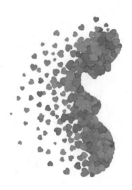

Notice to Readers

Laws are constantly changing. Every effort is made to keep this publication as current as possible. However, the author, the publisher, and the vendor of this book make no representations or warranties regarding the outcome or the use to which the information in this book is put and are not assuming any liability for any claims, losses, or damages arising out of the use of this book. The reader should not rely on the author or the publisher of this book for any professional advice. Please be sure that you have the most recent edition.

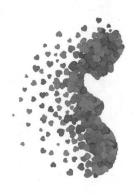

Dedication

This book is dedicated to all the moms who've spent part of their pregnancy lying down, patiently (and many times impatiently) incubating their baby, in hopes of reaching a magical milestone before delivering. It is also for the husbands, wives, partners, parents, siblings, children, friends, and medical support teams that play a role in supporting moms through this difficult journey.

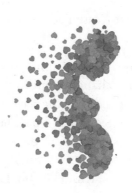

Acknowledgments

While there are many people who I would like to acknowledge, there isn't enough room here to thank everyone who helped me during my two bed rest pregnancies. My husband Kyle Yakimovitch was my rock and constant support. He never once complained about getting up at 4 a.m. to fill my cooler with food for my day on the couch, having to solo parent our daughter, or taking on all the household chores and responsibilities while I lied in bed. My parents Ken and Phyllis Lockrey put their lives on hold to help parent my daughter, Teagan, while I was living in the hospital.

I would also like to thank the many nurses, doctors, OBs, and other staff who played a role in the care and treatment of my children and me.

A special thank you to my obstetrician Dr. Renato Natale at London Health Sciences Centre. The first time I met Dr. Natale, he looked me in the eye and said, "Do you know why you are here? No doctor wants to treat you as your history scares them. You don't scare me." At that moment many of my fears were calmed. I loved his straightforward and honest approach. I'm so grateful to have had him as my OB. Even though my case had some twists and turns, he was always calm and focused.

To the moms on my antenatal unit: Thank you for the laughter, tears, and endless hours hanging out in the common room. Our time together not only helped pass the days as new friendships were formed, but also made me feel I was a part of a community, instead of being isolated in my room. The 56 days we spent together went by in a flash. Thank you to Nicole Bontaine, Jen van der Meulen, Lisa Gow, Katrina Greidanus, Laura Grubb, Deanna Cullen-Lawson, and Stephanie Keeping (our honorary mom). Although we now live on opposite sides of the country, I love staying connected and seeing pictures of your "babies" as they grow.

Finally, thank you to all my family and friends for your support. I hope this book will pay forward everything you have done to help my family and me in our bed rest journeys.

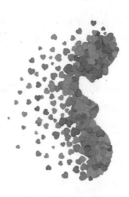

Preface

This book is not meant to offer medical advice, rather wisdom from the trenches from a mom who has spent her share of time on home- and hospital-based bed rest. The book contains tips and information on how not only I survived my bed rests, but also advice and stories from moms I've met along the way.

I decided to write this book after my son was born. Having had two pregnancies that involved prescribed bed rest — one at home and one in hospital — I have not known a "normal" pregnancy. In talking to other moms, I have learned there isn't much information out there for those of us who have been placed on bed rest, other than a couple of paragraphs in pregnancy books.

Much of the content comes from my own personal experience and the amazing people I encountered along the way. When I was pregnant with my daughter, at 22 weeks I was diagnosed with complete placenta previa, a condition where the placenta covers the cervix. In the majority of cases the placenta moves away from the cervix as the uterus grows. Not in my case. After some initial confusion and vague bed rest rules, I landed in hospital with minor bleeding at 28 weeks. Fortunately I lived within a three-minute drive from the hospital and was able to spend much of my time at home (with the occasional short-term stay each time I had a small bleed). Finally, at 36 weeks I delivered a small but healthy girl.

Fast-forward three years and I found out I was pregnant with my son. Although I was told each pregnancy is different, I strongly suspected more bed rest was in my future. I was right. My 20-week ultrasound revealed a suspected placenta accreta (when the placenta adheres to the muscle of the uterus or grows through the uterine wall versus attaching to its lining). I was sent to a high-risk hospital for further investigation where an ultrasound detected yet another complete placenta previa. Since I now lived 20 minutes from our small community hospital, which wasn't equipped to deal with placenta accreta, I was admitted to the antenatal unit of the regional teaching hospital more than an hour's drive from my home.

Although I'd never heard the term antenatal before, I settled in for my six-week stay on this high-risk unit with 20 other moms all trying their best to get close to their due date. I quickly made friends with a core group of moms who, like me, were in it for the long haul. We were a mixed bunch of shortened cervixes, placenta previas, low levels of amniotic fluids, gestational diabetes, and women carrying multiples. While we all had our own stories, we bonded over our love of daytime television, OREO cookies, and avoidance of Salisbury steak night.

As you find your own way to get through this challenging time in your life, I hope you gain your own insights from my experiences as well as those of the exceptional women who've had their own bed rest journeys.

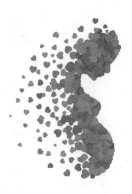

Introduction

Welcome to the world of bed rest. You have likely purchased or been given this book after receiving word from your obstetrician/gynecologist (OB/GYN)/doctor/midwife that you are being placed on bed rest. At first the idea of being given permission to rest, lie down, and relax seems pretty enticing. But depending on where you are in your pregnancy, your complications, whether you have other children to care for, and the restrictions placed on your bed rest, it can be a pretty daunting task.

The purpose of this book isn't to provide you with medical advice. Hopefully you've already established medical support to guide you through that portion of your pregnancy. Rather, this book is meant as a mom-to-mom resource to help guide you through your bed rest and provide you with some tips from moms who have been there.

Many women placed on bed rest have lots of questions and few people to talk to who understand their journey. Their friends all brag about how they worked until the day they delivered or tell stories of all the normal things they did during their pregnancy. This is not the case for women on bed rest. We are often left on our own to figure it out, with no one to talk to who truly understands what we are going through. It can be an isolating and lonely experience.

Hopefully the information contained in this book will help you prepare and make the best of your situation, whether at home or in the hospital.

The book is divided into two parts focusing on home-based bed rest and hospital-based bed rest. If you read the entire book, you will notice some duplication between the sections, as some information is the same regardless of where you spend your time. However, there are also many differences in resting at home versus being monitored in a hospital setting. Some women begin their bed rest at home but as their pregnancy progresses or complications arise, move into a hospital setting.

I encourage you to not only read the text but also complete the exercises in the book. These exercises are designed to get you thinking about some of the common challenges related to bed rest. They will help move you through this journey.

It is also important you write down and share any medical questions with your healthcare provider. Some of the information may get you thinking about what questions to ask, not only about your current situation, but also as you move closer to your due date and even after baby is born. Just as every pregnancy is different, each woman's bed rest, restrictions, and health issues before, during, and after pregnancy are also different.

Hopefully this book will help you realize you aren't alone. The stories from moms who have spent days and weeks on bed rest were written to help moms going through a similar journey as we all want our experiences to help other women. Please know there are many women who are cheering you on from the trenches. You are not alone.

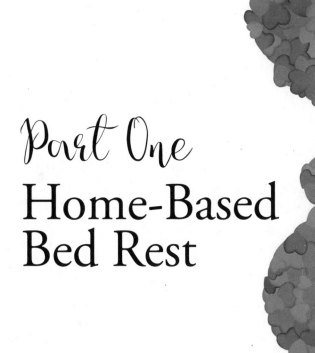

Part One
Home-Based Bed Rest

Before we get started, I want to share some points to help you navigate through the information contained in this book. Don't worry about keeping this book in pristine condition. Rather, I'd recommend you have a pen nearby so you can make notes, work through exercises, and jot down questions for both your medical and support teams.

You will notice there is some duplication of the information contained in the home-based and hospital-based bed rest sections (Parts I and II of this book). While it might be tempting to skip over the duplicated material, I would recommend taking the time to read the book in its entirety. There are some subtle and not-so-subtle differences between the two types of bed rest as the two forms are very different experiences.

As you read, take note of the information you need for your particular experience and ignore the rest.

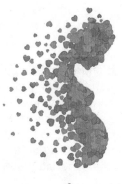

Chapter 1

Be Your
Own Advocate

While this entire book is about helping you care for yourself, both at home and in hospital, it begins with recognizing that as a person and as a patient you have rights. You have the right to know exactly what is happening to your body and details about your condition. You have the right to have this explained to you in a way that you will understand. You also have the right to ask questions and speak to someone else if you still are not satisfied with the information you are given. Your pregnancy is a time to advocate for yourself, and your baby, and not be a passive passenger in what can be a complex and emotional journey.

My pregnancy with my daughter happened three months after a devastating miscarriage at 11 weeks, 5 days. For anyone who has experienced a miscarriage, you understand why I remember how many days and weeks I was pregnant. For those of you who have been fortunate enough to have not suffered this loss, I share the following story not to scare you, but rather remind you of the importance of taking an active role in managing your pregnancy and bed rest.

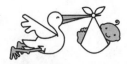

I had been so excited and optimistic about my first pregnancy, focusing on the baby and planning for the future, that I never thought for a second it would end in a miscarriage. To be honest, I had heard very little about miscarriages and had never known anyone who had miscarried (or so I thought). So when bleeding sent me to the doctor and then the hospital for an ultrasound, and I heard the news the baby had passed, my world fell apart.

What? How could this be? There must be some mistake. Sure, I was 35 years old, but my mother had children up until age 40, and I was in great health.

After taking some time to grieve, and much stress about the future, we got pregnant again. This time I was very guarded about my pregnancy, not sharing the news until I was well into the second trimester. I kept waiting for something to happen.

Living with this stress, and being on the other side of the country from my family, the first part of my pregnancy was a blur. Looking back, I think this is why I didn't advocate for myself or ask more questions. Instead I went to every appointment with my family doctor, happy to hear her say all was fine. Even when I was diagnosed with complete placenta previa at 22 weeks, I didn't get too upset or do my typical research. My doctor told me it wasn't a big deal and my placenta would likely move up as my uterus grew. Not wanting to think about any problems with my pregnancy, I believed it would all go away and I'd be fine. I was wrong.

My placenta never did move, rather it stubbornly remained over my cervix for the remainder of my pregnancy.

Despite my wanting to believe everything was okay, I had a nagging feeling something wasn't right. I was extremely drained. I was working a stressful full-time job, which I had only started two weeks before my miscarriage. I was in the stage of my new job where I was trying to prove myself, putting in long hours. I was working as the senior manager of media relations at a venue city for the Vancouver 2010 Winter Olympic Games. With the Olympics two years away, there wasn't time for me to fully process my loss or have the work/life balance a pregnant mom craves. Adding to that, my commute to work was 45 minutes to two hours, depending on traffic. My new job had required my husband and me to move across the country to a new community with few friends.

The combination of all these stresses was too much for me. I made an appointment with my family doctor and asked to be taken off work. Instead of being supportive, she lectured me about the importance of learning to juggle work and the demands of motherhood. I had already been diagnosed with placenta previa, which should have meant automatic bed rest.

My doctor thought this diagnosis was no big deal, as she was confident it would resolve itself. Even when I was later placed on full bed rest and transferred to the care of an obstetrician (OB) she still grumbled that she didn't see why all the fuss was being made about my pregnancy.

The first time I learned my placenta previa was a problem was when I'd gone to the hospital for suspected leaking fluids. The OB on call asked me how I got to the hospital. When I told him I'd driven myself he was shocked. He said I shouldn't be driving and should be on bed rest, but gave me limited information on what bed rest meant and my restrictions.

I begin the book with this story to show you that by not advocating for myself or really trying to understand my pregnancy and complications (my placenta previa), I put both my health and my baby at risk. Yes, I did ask to be taken off of work, but I didn't take the time to really understand the diagnosis of placenta previa, its complications, and restrictions. Instead, I trusted my doctor when she said it would resolve itself. Looking back, I should have asked to be transferred to an OB instead of staying with my family doctor. I had forgotten that patients in any healthcare system always have the right to ask to be referred to a specialist. Don't wait for your family doctor to refer you if you have concerns about your health and/or treatment. This is your body, and it is okay to take an active role in asking to see a specialist.

When I was pregnant with my son, I made sure I was referred to an OB the day I peed on the stick and found out I was pregnant.

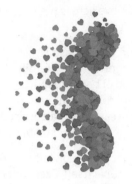

Chapter 2

Know the Rules: Types of Home-Based Bed Rest

The term "bed rest" is vague. Many women envision being confined to their bed until their baby is born, which, in reality, is the case for only a small percentage of moms. The restrictions placed on women who are put on bed rest are wide ranging and can vary throughout their pregnancies.

It is important to be clear on what type of bed rest you have been placed on and your specific restrictions. When I was originally placed on home bed rest after my first visit to the hospital, my only limitations were to keep trips up and down the stairs to a minimum, no working, as well as resting when I could. I was still allowed to go on light shopping trips or a coffee date with a friend.

This changed after a bleed that put me in the hospital for 72 hours. The OB on call was shocked that I had been shopping and dining with my husband instead of resting on the couch. She was furious my family doctor hadn't clearly spelled out the dangers associated with my condition and warned me that as the baby grew, so would the pressure on my cervix, which could in turn cause severe, and potentially life-threatening bleeding. My Saturday outing and associated walking had resulted in increased pressure on my cervix and a bleed that could have easily caused an early delivery.

I was terrified. At this point the OB was arranging for me to be flown to a hospital three hours away as there were no high-risk beds available in our area. I begged her to let me stay, promising not to bleed anymore (as if I had any control), and was told they would monitor me in the hospital for 72 hours. If the bleeding stopped, then I could go home. If the bleeding continued, I would spend the remainder of my pregnancy on bed rest in a hospital that could accommodate high-risk moms.

Thankfully, the bleeding stopped and I was allowed to go home. However, before being discharged, the OB sat on my bed and had a long discussion with me about bed rest, my limitations, and restrictions as they related to my condition, and what could happen to me and my baby if I didn't follow my bed rest rules.

I was then transferred to the care of an OB for the remainder of my pregnancy, so she could keep a close eye on me. On my weekly visits, my OB would review my symptoms, ask me about movements and, if there were no complications, allow me certain outings; car rides with my husband or ice cream at the beach. But each outing had to be within a short drive of the hospital and was for a set amount of time. Then it was back on the couch or to bed.

She was very clear in setting limits and letting me know that each outing needed to be preapproved by her. These outings were limited to once a week, sometimes once every two weeks.

Be careful about Googling the term "bed rest" or any of your medical conditions. It is too easy to pick the definition you prefer, telling yourself "well this is bed rest, so it must apply to me." Dr. Google can also cause unnecessary stress as there is the risk you will focus on the worst-case scenario versus the reality of your specific condition. Your medical provider knows you and your pregnancy best. It's important to have ongoing conversations with your medical provider with updates on your pregnancy, concerns, and energy levels, reviewing your bed rest restrictions to determine if any adjustments need to be made.

1. Questions to Ask Your Medical Team

See Exercise 1 for some common clarification questions to ask your medical provider about what bed rest means to your particular pregnancy and current condition.

Exercise 1
Questions to Ask Your Medical Team

Time off Feet

- Am I to be in bed and/or on the couch all day?

- May I walk for short periods of time? How long? How often?

- What distance (in the house, to the end of the driveway, around the block)?

- May I get up to go to the bathroom? Take showers? Baths? If so, for how long?

- May I go to the kitchen to make my meals?

- Am I allowed to take part in meal preparation or can I just grab items from the fridge?

Sitting versus Lying Down

- Am I allowed to sit up or do I need to lie down all the time?

- Do I need to lie on my side or can I lie on my back, slightly elevated?

- Do you want me to spend more time on my left side (often preferred)?

- If I can sit up, for how long?

- Can I eat meals at the table or do I need to be in bed or propped up on the couch?

Exercise 1 — Continued

Activities

- Can I drive myself to appointments? If so, is there a restriction on how far I can drive (ten minutes versus one hour)?

- Can I pick up my kids at school or drive them to their activities?

- Can I do prenatal yoga or other light stretching exercises? *If so, get specific instructions on what is allowed, with your caregiver showing you the recommended exercises so there is no confusion.*

- Can I get a massage or see a chiropractor? *If so, are there any restrictions (sometimes foot massages are off limits as they can induce labor).*

- Can I climb the stairs? If so, how many times a day?

- Can I lift things (my kids)? Weight limits?

Use the following table to make your own list of questions and discuss them with your healthcare provider. Then make a list of your restrictions, and review them each visit to see if any of the restrictions have changed. This is important, as your provider may not think to change restrictions based on changes in your pregnancy. It is up to you to be as open and honest about your situation, and take a proactive approach in continually reviewing your bed rest restrictions at each appointment.

Other Questions	Restrictions

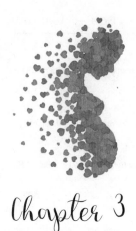

Chapter 3

What to Expect

So now, hopefully you're clear on what bed rest means to you. You have your list of restrictions, now what? If you only have a few days left in your pregnancy, well then kick your feet up and enjoy the last quiet moments before baby arrives. That is, if this is your first child. If you have other children, it's not so simple. You will need to reach out to your friends and family to get help caring for your children. The younger they are, the more help you are going to need … even if only for a few days.

However, if you have a week or more before your baby's birth, or even a few months, it's time to start thinking about what to do with yourself and the support your family will need to get through this challenging time. For those of you who don't have children at home, the first few days you will likely try to transition from working to bed rest, sleeping in, catching up on some television, and getting to that book you've been meaning to read. Once that is done, you'll soon find the days can be long to fill. For the moms with busy kids, you will need to figure out how you can parent from the couch, the support you and your family will need, and how to minimize the stress of this new reality for everyone. If you are a Type A personality, you can view bed rest as a project, one that requires careful planning.

Some of the items you will need to plan for include:

- Transitioning from work to bed rest.
- Finding support to help with your kids.
- Organizing your medical appointments.
- Developing a list of people you can call for rides and emergencies.
- Making a list of what you want to accomplish before baby arrives, including developing your birth plan.

The first step in getting organized for working moms is to find a way to finish up any loose ends at work (with your medical provider's permission) so you can turn your attention towards your baby. For moms with kids, you will need to hire a babysitter or have a friend watch the kids so you can make this transition as well as determine the help you and your family will need in the coming weeks (more about this in upcoming chapters).

If your kids are not in school or daycare, think about how you will keep them busy during the day, as you won't be able to chase after your toddler or prevent him or her from making a mess in the bathroom. You won't be able to relax and get the rest your body needs if you have young children running around without some help.

The next step in getting organized is entering all your medical appointments into the calendar. If your restrictions prevent you from driving, you will need to schedule transportation for your appointments. It is also handy to create an in-case of emergency list that is near you at all times. Who can drive you to the hospital if needed? Who can come and quickly take care of your kids? Your pet? Planning in advance can relieve some stress as you know you're prepared if an emergency arises — even if you never have to use your list. See Exercise 2.

When I was on home-based bed rest, my husband worked two hours away. In the early days of bed rest I didn't have an emergency contact list, as I didn't think anything would happen to me. I had pre-arranged that my real estate agent (who had become a friend) would drive me to my weekly OB appointments.

Exercise 2
Develop Your On-Call List

The length of your on-call list of people you will need to support you and your family, and number of areas you will need support will depend on how much longer you have in your pregnancy.

The purpose of this exercise is to help you create your on-call list of family and friends that are available to drive you to appointments and come at a moment's notice during emergencies.

Here are some questions to ask as you develop your on-call list.

Emergencies

- Who can get to your house in less than 10 minutes? Less than 30 minutes?
- How far do you live from the hospital?
- What is the most direct route?
- What floor is the maternity unit at the hospital? Make sure your driver knows to take you to the maternity floor not the emergency room (and confirm this is correct with your medical provider).

Medical appointments

- List all of your medical appointments including date, time, location, reason.
- How long is each appointment?
- Does your driver need to stay with you or can he or she drop you off and pick you up when you're ready?
- Do you need a wheelchair to get from the car to the appointment? If so, is there a wheelchair available at the appointment, and where should your driver go to get the wheelchair?

Considering all the questions you've answered above, fill out the following tables to help you organize your appointments as well as people who are available to drive you to appointments or help during an emergency.

Rides to medical appointments					
Date	Time	Location	Appointment	Driver	Special instructions

On-call driver list				
Less than 10 minutes away				
Name	Phone number	Email	Days and times available	Available for emergencies?

Less than 30 minutes away				
Name	**Phone number**	**Email**	**Days and times available**	**Available for emergencies?**

One day I had some light spotting/bleeding and I panicked. I called my husband, who said even if he left immediately, with rush hour traffic it would take him two hours to get home. He was worried the spotting would lead to major bleeding, and told me I needed to go to the hospital immediately. He would meet me there.

I agreed. In my panic I never thought to call an ambulance. So I called our real estate agent (who at this point had only driven me to two appointments and I was still getting to know). Not only did she drive me to the hospital, but she also insisted on staying with me until the OB had seen me and determined the next steps. Since my friend was much older than me, the nurse assumed she was my mother and went on to have a very personal discussion about bleeding and discharge with my friend sitting at my bedside. Since she didn't seem uncomfortable, and I really wanted someone to be with me, she sat through the nurse helping me change into a gown (moms soon learn to not be modest), and me cringing while the IV was inserted. She kept me distracted until the OB arrived. Thankfully she excused herself for the examination. I was grateful that she dropped everything to come get me and take me to the hospital. More importantly, that she stayed and kept me calm until my husband arrived.

After this trip, I made some phone calls to determine who was available to drive me to the hospital during the day at a moment's notice. I had a list of drivers for different timeslots and on different days. My real estate friend had put her entire office on call to drive me to the hospital. They were given instructions on where I lived, what floor the maternity unit was on, and an overview of my condition. Yes, a bit much, but one of her coworkers ended up taking me to a medical appointment when my friend was called out to meet with a prospective buyer. Since they had been briefed on my situation, her coworker was more than happy to fill in. She was an extremely pleasant woman who had also been on bed rest with one of her children. We had lots to talk about during the ride.

In developing my on-call list I ended up making new friends, which was extremely important as I had just moved to the community a few months earlier. It also served as an ice-breaker for the women in my prenatal class, as some of them became my chauffeurs, with their own schedule of who was driving me where and when, as I also had to have blood taken every three days at the hospital (to cross match in case I needed a blood transfusion).

The final step is making a list of what you want to accomplish before your baby arrives. A good first start is to think about your baby's birth and developing a birth plan. Even if you don't think you are going to be spending your pregnancy in hospital, I would recommend reading Chapter 20 where I explain how a birth plan for high-risk pregnancy is different from our low-risk counterparts. There is also an exercise on items to include in your birth plan.

Is there a photo book you want to complete? A book series you've always wanted to read? A hobby you want to take up or master — such as knitting, painting, or jewelry making? Daycare applications you want to fill out? Summer camps or extracurricular activities you want to register your children for? It's a good idea to list what interests you and think about how you can advance those interests from your bed. Also, are there activities you can safely do from your bed or couch?

There can be great satisfaction in working on a hobby or project you can grow and develop, much like the baby incubating inside you. I know one mom who not only learned how to knit, but ended up knitting baby hats for all of her friends on her floor in the hospital. She said the baby hats not only took less time to make than larger projects, such as a blanket, but she also had the gratification of handing out the hats to her friends to help them focus on the babies they were growing.

If crafts don't interest you, and you're say, a marathon runner, you can research running tips, set up a post-pregnancy nutrition program, or investigate marathons you'd like to eventually run. If you're a writer, now's the time to pull out the laptop and begin working on that blog, website, article, or book. Unless you have children at home, you'll have minimal distractions and can focus on your writing. The idea is to fulfill your passions and spend this time filling your bucket versus emptying it in boredom.

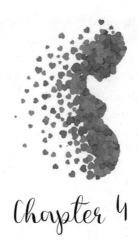

Chapter 4

Importance of Routine for At-Home Bed Rest

Even though your days on bed rest are spent inside your home, it is still important to establish a regular routine. Sure, this won't look anything like your "normal life" routine, but it will help you feel normal.

Why should you bother? If you don't set a routine, the days can seem endless and you will quickly get bored. While it might look great at first to have no plans, it won't take long before you are ready to climb the walls.

Think about this: In your normal life you have a somewhat set schedule of when you get up, when you eat your meals, and what activities you do at what time. Sure this schedule may vary a bit from day to day, but there is still some structure to your days. Trust me, it is this structure that not only helps us know what to expect but also helps us feel balanced throughout the day.

What an average day looks like for a mom on bed rest depends on the individual. Establishing a schedule helps to divide your day into blocks of time, as sitting in front of the TV for 12 hours can be depressing. Instead, try to stimulate your mind with different activities.

There is an upcoming exercise to help you explore how to plan your day. Before you do the exercise, here are some ideas on what an average day can look like.

Plan to get up roughly the same time every day. If you're tired, sleep in, but if not, get out of bed and start your day. Have your shower after getting up (if allowed) then have breakfast, as pregnant women cannot go long without food.

You might want to spend an hour or so in the morning watching TV while you eat your breakfast. Then turn it off, and read a book or work on your laptop until lunch. Have your lunch with a friend at your house or watch a favorite show. After lunch, take a nap or lie down to rest. Make sure your schedule sets aside time for naps, even short ones, as these not only shorten the days but also provide much needed rest for your growing body.

After your nap, you can work on one of the hobbies discussed earlier. Set aside a time to talk to friends on the phone. This way they know when is a good time to call and won't avoid calling you so they don't wake you from a nap (which can mean no one calls, furthering your feelings of isolation). You don't need to adhere firmly to your schedule, but it will help you feel as though you have some structure in your days.

Here's roughly what my schedule looked like during my home-based bed rest:

9:00 a.m.:	wake up, shower, get dressed
9:30 a.m.:	move to the couch
9:40 a.m.:	breakfast and morning television
11:00 a.m.:	read a book
12:00 p.m.:	lunch watching TV series on Netflix
1:00 p.m.:	nap
2:00 p.m.:	do some consulting work — writing, researching (a friend supplied me with work that wasn't time sensitive and I could do from the couch)

4:00 p.m.:	phone calls with friends/family
5:00 p.m.:	read a book
6:00 p.m.:	supper with my husband or a friend (on the couch)
7:00 p.m.:	phone calls with friends/family
8:00 p.m.:	TV with my husband
10:00 p.m.:	bedtime

This routine really helped me fill the days and feel like I had accomplished something. By structuring my days in blocks, I had some variety. Sure, some days I was so engrossed in a book I spent the afternoon reading. Or, a friend would come over for a visit. But the key was variety. Too much of anything becomes monotonous.

Earlier in my pregnancy I had enrolled in a prenatal class that was being held at the hospital where I was to give birth. I had to pretty much beg my OB to let me attend, which she only agreed to because one of the maternity floor nurses was teaching the course. One of the conditions of me attending was I had to be in a wheelchair from the time I got out of my car until the time the class ended and I was back in my car.

That first class I was very self-conscious of being in a wheelchair. The nurse, who had been briefed on my condition by my OB, privately asked me if I wanted to share why I was on bed rest. I was tempted to say no, and try to hide away in the corner, but thought since everyone was a stranger, why not. Being vulnerable and talking about my experience was a turning point in my bed rest. Slowly the other women opened up about their pregnancies, and I realized no one has a "normal pregnancy." Everyone has challenges. That's the nature of pregnancy.

Many of the women in the room were also living far away from family. After week three of our prenatal class, some of the ladies who were off work or on limited work schedules (some due to their own pregnancy complications), decided to come for lunch at my house to keep me company. It was at this lunch, that I opened up about my struggles with bed rest, and increasing amount of appointments (even though I was supposed to be resting). After hearing about my challenges the moms created the chart I previously mentioned to drive me to my appointments. They were very happy to help in any way possible.

We also decided to have weekly potluck lunches at my house until my planned c-section date. As we all moved along in our pregnancies, the number of moms attending our lunches also grew in size, with eventually eight of the nine moms in our class coming to the weekly get-togethers. The lunches became half-day affairs, and we were grateful to spend time with other women at the same stage of pregnancy.

This weekly lunch date became an important part of my routine. My husband also took advantage of these days to work late or run errands, as he knew I was well fed and wasn't sitting at home alone waiting for him to come through the door.

Once the babies began entering the world, we would all gather to meet the new addition in the hospital. When my daughter was born, I had a private room (out of kindness from the nurses who had gotten to know me during my various admissions). I remember the nurse opening my room door and all of the women from my prenatal class were crammed into my small room; some with babies in arms and some with big bellies. We were laughing a bit too loudly.

The nurse had come to tell me I had too many visitors, but when she realized the women in the room were the women who had supported me throughout my pregnancy, through the good and the bad, she told us to have fun and closed the door.

After our babies we born, we continued our weekly lunches, rotating between each other's homes. This group shared breastfeeding challenges, asked each other questions about the color of our babies' poo (you talk a lot about poo in the early days) and became a great resource and support system to lean on. We had an amazing first birthday party for our babies, full of celebration for not only the babies, but also for us parents surviving the first year together.

Our children are now in school but we still keep in touch. It has been amazing to watch the children grow and know that our friendship all started because these women wanted to keep me company as I spent my pregnancy on bed rest.

The point of this story is you never know what new experiences await you, even when you are confined to a couch or a bed. Be open. If I hadn't have begged my OB to let me take the prenatal class, and instead resigned myself to staying home, I would have missed out on building this incredible support system with life-long friendships. I also added a new routine to my bed rest calendar: A weekly afternoon gathering with some amazing women.

Having hour upon hour of free, unstructured time may seem a blessing right now — well that is if you're not a Type A personality who loves to plan. If you enjoy this unstructured time, soak it up now. It won't take long before the lack of routine can cause boredom, and even depression.

To keep your spirits up and sanity intact, I'd strongly recommend taking some time to visualize your average day (I say average as we are thinking of a day that is free of medical appointments … just lying on the couch or in bed). For the days with medical appointments, you would adjust this schedule accordingly, but for the most part the routine would stay the same. (See Exercise 3.)

Exercise 3
Planning Your Day

This exercise will lead you through some questions to ask yourself to help you create a schedule that works for you and your family.

- When are you most alert? Morning, afternoon, or evening?

- If you have no interruptions or planned activities, when does your body naturally wake up?

- What is your morning routine? Example: shower first, then breakfast, then checking social media, then getting kids ready. Be as specific as possible on what your first hour typically looks like.

- If applicable, what time does your partner leave for work?

- If you have kids, what time do they leave for daycare/school/work?

- Do you have any regular appointments? If so, what time are they and on what day(s)?

- What books do you want to read? Is there a particular series you want to read? (This will also help you create a wish list for friends to pick up books from the library for you.)

- What TV shows or movies do you want to watch?

- Do you have a hobby you enjoy that you can do from the couch or bed? Examples: knitting, painting, jewelry making, genealogy.

- Is there a hobby you would like to learn?

- What are some of your favorite activities when you don't have restrictions? Examples: yoga, running, hiking, team sports, art.

- What would you like to learn more about your favorite activity (think what can you research from the couch)?

- Is there an online course or certification you would like to take?

- What time do you normally eat breakfast?

  - Lunch?

  - Supper?

- What are your favorite snacks?

- What friends and family can come for a visit?

- When is the best time for them to visit? During the day? After work?

This is just a starter list of questions to get you thinking about your day. Feel free to jot down anything else you envision yourself doing during your time at home. Obviously your routine may vary from day to day based on appointments and visitors. But visualizing your typical day will help you know what your days will look like and help you find activities that stimulate versus bore you to fill in the time.

Now, looking at your answers above, plot your typical day. This is a great exercise to share with your partner and/or children so they have an idea of what you have planned. It will help them know when you want some alone time or a nap and when you are looking for company.

6:00 a.m.	
7:00 a.m.	
8:00 a.m.	
9:00 a.m.	
10:00 a.m.	
11:00 a.m.	
12:00 p.m.	
1:00 p.m.	
2:00 p.m.	
3:00 p.m.	
4:00 p.m.	
5:00 p.m.	
6:00 p.m.	
7:00 p.m.	
8:00 p.m.	
9:00 p.m.	
10:00 p.m.	
11:00 p.m.	

Laura's Story

Laura Grubb
Mother of two
Sixteen weeks of hospital-based bed rest

Bed rest can be a blessing if you allow it to be. You are not likely to ever again have people deliver your meals, clean your living space, and shoulder your responsibilities. Accept that things will not always be to your liking, the food may be bland, and tasks not completed to your standard. I know because my son was wearing his winter boots well into summer before it occurred to anyone to get him some running shoes.

Life moves on. Looking back, those moments are funny memories of an abnormal time. Appreciate that others are there to step in, especially if you have children. Remember that sometimes being a parent or a sibling means sacrificing to put someone else first. In bed rest, your unborn child is being put first.

However, bed rest is not easy. Being separated from loved ones during such a time of incredible worry is difficult. Talk to others, cry, and take a day to feel sad; these are all OK. I used to lock the door to the bathroom in my room for privacy during days when I needed to release the stress of worrying about my high-risk pregnancy without intrusion.

Fill your days with routine as much as possible. Find a productive activity that will fulfill your need to do something. Organize your family photos, read a whole series of books you have not gotten around to reading, or craft something special.

Be sure to ask about your limitations. If you are permitted to go for a walk, get out of your room and meet other moms. Building a network of other moms, who are also on bed rest, will provide you with a wealth of support, not to mention help the time pass faster.

Stay focused on the positive during your bed rest. Take time to lie down and savor the feeling of your baby moving each morning. Every night be thankful for another day of growth and health for your baby. Let each day be a mini-celebration of your baby's growth and maturing.

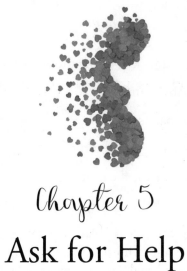

Chapter 5

Ask for Help

Once word gets out you've been put on bed rest, you will have friends, family, and neighbors saying "let me know if there is anything I can do to help." You'll likely brush away these offers, saying you're fine. After all, they're just saying that to be polite. Wrong.

Don't guess at others' intentions. By accepting support and asking for help you'll soon find out who is sincere in wanting to support you during this challenging time. This is a time when you truly need that help. However, before you ask for help, be clear on what specific help you and your family need.

Here's a list of some areas in which you might need help during your bed rest days:

- Rides to your appointments

- Rides for your children

- Meals and snacks for you and your family

- House cleaning

- Laundry

- Grocery shopping

- Haircuts

- Pedicures (good luck reaching those toes)

- Setting up baby's nursery

- Shopping for baby's arrival

- Picking up relatives at the airport

- Packing your bag for the hospital

- Setting up your baby registry

Asking for help can feel awkward. It's tough to know who is sincere about an offer and who isn't. Here's a tip I used when I was placed on home-based bed rest. I sent an email to friends, family, and coworkers providing an update on my pregnancy. Since I had been placed on bed rest with no warning, I never had a chance to say goodbye to my coworkers or let friends know in advance that I would spend the remainder of my pregnancy on the couch. In the email I clearly listed the help I needed. This was less awkward for me as I wasn't directly asking anyone for help, so no one felt obligated. By being specific through a general email about how people could help me, it let my friends and family know my needs and allowed them to respond accordingly, with no awkward conversations.

The response was overwhelming and help came from the most unlikely places. The real estate agent who helped us buy our house signed up to drive me to all my OB appointments. A work colleague I didn't know well, but soon came to cherish, came by every Tuesday night with a hot meal — providing much needed company for me as well as a break for my husband. She also brought movies, books, and updates from the office. Others dropped off meals, stopped by for tea, or bought groceries for us. One friend, who was busy running her own business, bought me eight hours of house cleaning through a service. She felt bad that she couldn't help personally, but found her own way to take some of the stress off my husband and me. Yet another friend picked us up supper items at her weekly Costco shop. She enjoyed picking out different entrees each week, getting one for us and one for her family. She said it encouraged her to try something different each week.

You may want to find your own way to ask for help — but make sure you are as clear as possible about your needs. Don't brush off offers from friends and family. This is the time you truly need to rely on your social network. By asking for specific help, this network can help you in the way that works best for them. And you won't end up with a freezer full of tuna casseroles.

Asking for help can be hard for many women. For this reason, I want to push you out of your comfort zone and have you spend time being clear on what help you truly need and how your friends/family can best support you.

My hope is that by doing Exercise 4 you will take the time to really reflect on your current situation and your personal and family needs. When you've completed the exercise, please share this information with your family and friends who want to support you but don't know how.

The table in Exercise 4 will help you visualize how the people in your life can help you in a variety of ways. You can also put this chart on the fridge so you and your family know who to call for specific help.

Once you've done that, you'll need to ask for help in a clear and specific way. How you do this can vary on your relationships. You can send a mass email to all of your friends/family/coworkers using the template in Example 1 or you can have individual conversations using Exercise 4 as a tool on what your specific needs are — both now and after baby is born. What is important is that you are specific on the support you need and your family needs and how each person can help.

Exercise 4
Asking for Help from Family and Friends

What are your current bed rest limitations? Check all that apply.

[   ]   No stairs

[   ]   No standing

[   ]   Standing for a limit of _____ minutes

[   ]   No driving

[   ]   No lifting

[   ]   No meal preparation

[   ]   No shopping

[   ]   No laundry

[   ]   No or limited cleaning

[   ]   Limited self care (bathing, dressing)

[   ]   Fully confined to bed

[   ]   Other _____

How many hours a day are you confined to the bed and/or couch?

How many medical appointments do you have each week and the length of each appointment?

[   ]   OB

[   ]   Blood tests

[   ]   Physiotherapy

[   ]   Naturopath

[   ]   Chiropractor

[   ]   Massage therapy

[   ]   Other _____

If you have children at home, what are your current and future limitations in caring for your children?

What activities are your children involved in which require support? Examples: tutoring, sports, clubs, school. Be specific on times, dates, locations.

Who typically prepares the meals in your family?

How are meals currently being prepared for you and your family?

What types of meals does your family enjoy?

If friends were to provide food, what is the best way of helping you in meal preparation? Example: already prepared meals that just require heating or preportioned and chopped ingredients for a family member to put together (e.g., fixings for tacos or stir-fry). Be clear on what foods your family likes as well as any food allergies, sensitivities, or dislikes. It's important to state what your family won't eat so none of the food is wasted.

What support do you need inside of the home?

[   ]   Cleaning

[   ]   Laundry

[   ]   Meal preparation

[   ]   Personal care

[   ]   Organizing baby's room

[   ]   Visits to keep you company

[   ]   Other _____

What support do you need for your children?

[   ]   Homework support

[   ]   Play dates or babysitting

[   ]   Bath care

[   ]   Bedtime

[   ]   Lunches

[   ]   Other _____

What support do you need outside of the home?

[   ]   Grocery shopping – taking you

[   ]   Grocery shopping – doing it for you

[   ]   Dropping off/picking up children from school/daycare

[   ]   Shuttling children to extracurricular activities

[   ]   Other _____

What friends/family/coworkers have offered support (the "let me know if you need anything" statement)? Also include anyone you know who could offer support both locally and remote.

What are your greatest stresses?

How many days/weeks are left until your due date?

Now review the questions and, in a different color pen, answer the same questions based on your anticipated needs after baby is born. Remember: Often women who have been on bed rest have a harder time "bouncing back" versus women who have been mobile throughout their pregnancy. This is often due to muscle atrophy and other pregnancy complications.

Exercise 4 — Continued

The next step is to review your answers and fill out the chart below.

The column on the left is support needed. In the top row fill in the names of friends and family members who can help, checking the appropriate support they can provide based on your relationship and comfort level. I've left room for other forms of support.

SUPPORT NEEDED							
Inside the home							
Meal prep							
Cleaning							
Organizing baby's room							
Laundry							
Personal care							
Packing your hospital bag							
Outside the home							
Shopping							
Groceries							
Rides to appointments							
Pickups at airport							
For the children							
Homework support							
Rides to activities							
Play dates or babysitting							
Lunch preparation							
Getting on/off the bus							
Bath care							
Bedtime							

Example 1
Draft Email to Family and Friends

Hi family and friends,

I'm sorry for this group email, but I've found this is the best way to communicate and provide an update on my pregnancy. As many of you know, I've been put on bed rest for my health and my baby's health. While some people may view bed rest as a great excuse to lie back and relax until baby is born, I have to admit this is a very stressful time for my family and me. The limitations put on me mean I'm not able to do all the things that need to be done.

Some of you have offered your help, which is greatly appreciated. Instead of putting anyone on the spot, I thought it would be best to send a group email letting everyone know what support I need so you can decide how, if at all, you can help.

What I need help with includes:
[edit this list to suit your needs]

In the home

- Laundry
- Cleaning
- Meal preparation (either helping at meal time or supplying healthy prepared meals)
  [Be specific here on what you and your family like and don't like]
- Organizing baby's room
- Visits and keeping me company

For the children

- Homework support
- Play dates/babysitting
- Bath care
- Bedtime

Outside the home

- Rides to medical and personal appointments *[list dates and times if you have them]*
- Grocery shopping – driving and helping shop
- Grocery shopping – getting the list and the shopping
- Dropping off/picking up children from school/daycare *[be specific on times/locations]*
- Shuttling children to extracurricular activities *[be specific on dates/times/locations]*

I'm hoping this list will help you better understand the support my family and I need. I'm happy for any help you can give.

I will continue to update you on this journey and thank each of you for all your love and support.

[Your name]

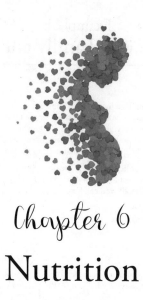

Chapter 6

Nutrition

Eating is an important topic for pregnant women. When I was pregnant I could never go more than a couple of hours without food. While snacking is a normal part of pregnancy, it can be a bit tricky when you're on bed rest.

Just as it is important to plan your activities for the day, it's also important to plan your food in advance. Depending on your bed rest restrictions, you may not be able to go grocery shopping or even walk to the kitchen to prepare a snack. Some women are limited in how long they can stand each hour, having to choose between going to the bathroom or going to the fridge.

Bed rest is the time to bring out the camping cooler. A great trick is to have your partner fill the cooler with snacks and meals. It's also good to have a box with nonperishable snacks (e.g., crackers, nuts, seeds, granola bars) next to your bed and next to you on the couch.

My husband was in charge of food preparation. Each morning he filled a cooler with a mixture of fruits, vegetables, yogurt, sandwiches, cottage cheese, and other goodies to get me through the day until he came home from work for supper. He removed a cushion from our sectional couch and placed the cooler next to where I'd be resting.

Then when I came downstairs in the morning I simply needed to open the cooler to get a bite to eat. It was like having a picnic on the couch.

One advantage to this method of having your day's nutrition prepared in advance, it helps to make sure you are getting food from each of the food groups. I found it was much easier to eat healthy as my husband only put healthy food in the cooler. The one drawback was when I had a craving for something that wasn't in my cooler — and we all know about pregnant women and their cravings. My solution when a craving struck was to go back to my previous point about asking for help. I had a friend who worked near an amazing cupcake store. Thankfully he was receptive to my urgent texts and would bring me mixed packages of mini cupcakes on his way home from work. The moms from my prenatal class, who were very familiar with pregnancy cravings, were also willing to bring me ice cream, a milkshake, or any other foods that I craved. These craving errands often ended up with us spending hours chatting or watching a movie together. It was a great way to have impromptu visits while my husband was at work.

While your restrictions may not allow you to go grocery shopping, thanks to the Internet, there are still many ways to get healthy food delivered to your home. Check and see if your local grocery store delivers. Some larger cities also have companies that deliver organic produce, prepared meals, and health products weekly.

Also research local restaurants and caterers who can supply you with healthy meals. Usually caterers are a better option, as they can custom make meals, providing either fresh meals or a selection of frozen entrees. By working with a caterer you can also be specific about ingredients used, which is especially helpful if you're on a special diet. You can also see if the caterer will deliver to your home, saving a trip for your partner, who is likely already loaded with extra chores.

I was able to connect with the owner of a local small restaurant and have her specially prepare meals for me. I had called the restaurant and told the owner my story about being on bed rest. She was very empathetic and asked me questions about what type of food my husband and I liked to eat, and any restrictions. She explained that she made all of her soups and meals from scratch with local ingredients, many grown in her garden. She offered to set aside portions of her soup each day and freeze them for me. On Saturdays, my husband would go to the restaurant and pick up the frozen portions. The soup I didn't eat during my bed rest made for easy lunches after my daughter was born. I also developed a new friend through this experience, as the owner asked us to bring our daughter in after she was born, as she felt invested in my pregnancy. Her restaurant became a regular stop while we were out shopping.

If you are buying prepared meals from grocery stores, make sure you read the ingredient list, choosing meals with real ingredients and passing on the preservatives and chemicals. If you're ordering from a restaurant, do your research. Pregnancy is an important time to eat fresh, healthy meals, not meals with a list of ingredients you can't pronounce. Smaller, local restaurants are often more willing to take the time to discuss ingredients and offer suggestions for healthy takeout dishes.

By planning your meals in advance, you will avoid falling into the trap of eating quick and convenient takeout meals, which are often void of any nutritional value. You should also consider stockpiling some frozen meals from your caterer for when baby is born as the first three months can be challenging as you all try to find a schedule and balance. Being on bed rest, unfortunately you won't have the chance to nest or fill the freezer with homemade meals and snacks. This is a great way to fulfill the nesting instinct, without all the hard work.

In the Appendix, I have listed some recommended books for healthy meals in pregnancy and beyond.

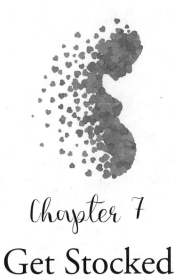

Chapter 7

Get Stocked

1. Bedroom Supplies

For most home-based bed rests, you'll likely break up your day by spending half your time in bed and half your time on the couch. However, those on more restrictive bed rest may spend the remainder of their pregnancy in bed.

Since it will be hard for you to get anywhere, here are some supplies you should have in your bedroom to keep you occupied for 12+ hours a day:

- Phone (landline; ideally not cordless)

- Cell phone charger

- Clock

- List of emergency contacts

- Books and/or magazines

- Pen and paper

- Checkbook (I will discuss this more later on)
- Lip balm
- Water bottle
- Nonperishable snacks (discussed more in section 2.)
- Flashlight with good batteries

Don't worry; while your bedroom will resemble a student dorm room, after baby is born, it will take on a new look: that of a second nursery.

2. Snacks

Oh, snacks, an important topic for all pregnant women. You don't want to be without food when the need for snacking hits. It's a good idea to fill a plastic storage container with nonperishable snacks and place it next to your bed. Once again, try to think healthy. If it's not in the container, you won't be eating it. Stick to food that provides the nutrition you need, with a few essential treats such as chocolate to enjoy.

Protein will help fill you more than carbohydrates. A great snack is homemade trail mix — nuts, seeds and, of course, chocolate. My favorite trail mix was a mix of almonds, walnuts, sunflower seeds, pumpkin seeds, cut up dates, and chunks of dark chocolate. A handful helped fill me until the next snack.

Other great items are granola bars (Cliff or Luna versus the traditional sugar-filled ones from the grocery store), crackers, mints (in case company is coming and you can't make it to the bathroom), and water: lots of water. Throw in some fruit that doesn't need refrigeration, such as apples, oranges, and bananas.

If you're fortunate enough to have a small fridge, you can fill it with milk, yogurt, and fruit salad. Maybe even a couple frozen treats.

These bedroom snacks will continue to be helpful for those late night or early morning feedings when baby comes home.

3. Entertainment

As mentioned earlier, you'll need a variety of activities to pass the time. In my experience, watching too much television can actually make the days seem longer. Instead, break it up with a combination of books, crafts, and screen time.

A television or laptop computer is an important feature of your entertainment collection. Watching a movie in bed can be a good way to pass the time. A Netflix or Apple TV subscription will ensure you don't run out of things to watch.

Depending on the length of your anticipated bed rest, now is a great time to watch a television series you've always found interesting. Netflix has no shortage of TV series. You can also check your local library for free rentals of movies and TV series. If you don't finish the series before baby comes, not to worry, you can continue watching it during those middle of the night feedings.

Make sure you also have a good book (or several) beside your bed. You might want to get a mix of educational books (related to your occupation, or baby guides) as well as books for entertainment. Once again, this is a great time to read or reread a series such as *Harry Potter, Twilight, Outlander, Hunger Games*, or *A Song of Ice and Fire*. Since pregnancy is a time of hormones, and the occasional mood swing, try to avoid books that are too heavy or deal with issues you find disturbing (with you *Game of Thrones/Ice and Fire* fans likely being the exception). Fantasy or romance novels were a better fit for me, while some women may prefer reading biographies or history books. This is also a good place to store your baby names book, as you'll have lots of time to test out different names, and drive your partner crazy asking what he or she thinks of this name or that name. Whatever your preference, you now have time to put up your feet and read a good book.

Make sure you have a journal and a pen in your bedroom. You may want to record your days, write notes to your child, or simply have a piece of paper to write down your grocery list. You know how you often cannot find a piece of paper when you need it; now imagine being confined to your bed and needing to write something down in a hurry. You will thank me for the reminder of having a journal (so you don't lose little scraps of paper) and a pen.

If you're interested in crafts, it's a good idea to have a container at your bedside with your craft supplies. This can be the same container from the couch so you can continue working on the same project(s), or a new container for a project you just work on from your bed. This container could include items for scrapbooking, knitting, or drawing. One good bedroom-based craft is a vision board. This will help you focus on the future you want for you and your family. The kit is pretty easy to assemble. Grab some old magazines, tape, glue, scissors, and get a piece of cardboard or foam core. Each day you can cut out words or pictures that resonate with you, slowly adding them to your vision board. At the end of the process, you will have a positive image to look at while in bed that reflects the future you desire, to help you focus on your future versus your current state of bed rest. It could be a good reminder of why you are doing all this hard work.

4. Sleep Essentials

If you're going to spend a lot of time lying down, you might as well get comfortable. Most pregnant women find a pregnancy-specific body pillow to be their best friend. Often these look like a six-foot tall "C." The idea is you rest your head on the top part of the "C," wrap your body and belly around the long part, putting it between your knees to relieve pressure from your back, and rest your feet on the bottom part. One common brand you can get in baby stores or online is called the Snoogle total body pillow. It helps remove pressure from your hips and lower back.

After baby is born you can use this pillow for baby's tummy time, as a breastfeeding pillow and, later, as support when the baby is sitting. I still have my pillow from my first pregnancy, although my husband confiscates it some nights.

You will also need to have a good selection of blankets that you can take off and put on as your body heats up and cools off. To keep a happy relationship with your partner, it's a good idea to have your own blankets at easy access on your side of the bed, so your partner doesn't end up suffering from your temperature adjustments.

Think of any other items you need for a good night (or day's) sleep. Are you someone who loves to be surrounded by pillows? Do you need a fan to keep the room cool? How about a nightlight to help with the middle of the night bathroom trips? Make a list of all the items you need to help you sleep. The further you are in your pregnancy, the more challenging it can be to get a good night's sleep, so you will need all the help you can get.

5. Other Bedroom Essentials

Also make sure your phone is within reach. I recommend you set up a landline with a non-cordless phone next to your bed (yes I know this sounds old-school but trust me: This way if the power goes out you will still be able to make phone calls and not worry if your cell or cordless phone is charged). There's a reason you are on bed rest, and you want to make sure you always have a phone near you in case you need to call for help.

Finally, it is important to have a few checks in your bedroom. Remember all those friends and family who are going to help you? Well it gets pretty awkward if you can't pay them for picking up your groceries. You can use email money transfers from your banking website for payment. This way you can keep track of who you paid and how much and won't need to worry about sending someone to the bank for you.

6. Living Room Essentials

You've showered, dressed, and have made it to the couch. Congratulations! Now how do you pass the next 12 hours? You'll want a duplication of many of the supplies we mentioned for your bedroom next to you on the couch. Notice I said "duplication" rather than suggest you carry everything from one location to the next. Not a good idea. It's best to have each area independently stocked. Unless you're completely engrossed in a particular book, you can have couch books, and bedroom books, giving you something to look forward to when you change locations.

A television, laptop, or tablet and access to movies is also essential from the couch; possibly even some video games. I was never a fan of video games until week three of bed rest. By then I had read more than 20 books, watched too many talk shows, and was bored of watching movies. A friend lent me his Xbox, loaded with games he thought I'd like — more puzzle than shoot-up. After two weeks of playing one puzzle game, I managed to get the top score, beating my friend who had a few more years of experience. I was pretty proud of myself and we bonded over game strategy.

I also enjoyed puzzle books; scrabble, word searches and the like. Once again, it gave me a break from my usual routine and a chance to use my brain. Trust me, it can be a welcome relief to use your brain after a few days or weeks of lying down.

You can also investigate some work-related activities that are low stress. I've had friends who took online courses, did consulting, or researched new business ideas from the couch. Remember, once baby arrives your energy will be consumed by your new love. So now is a good time to do the things you've been meaning to do but have never had the time. Just make sure it isn't too stressful or time sensitive, as your situation can change at a moment's notice.

I had a friend who would send me writing assignments that had long deadlines. I ended up writing website copy for one of her clients. This was a great assignment as I was able to slowly work away at developing various pages. If I hadn't been able to finish it, someone else could have picked up where I left off.

Finally, don't forget that cooler of food I mentioned earlier. It's amazing how hungry you can get, even though you don't think you're being active. Growing a baby is a lot of work and your body is using up considerable amounts of energy. Don't forget to eat.

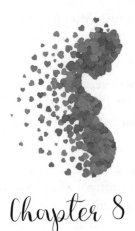

Chapter 8

Care for Your Body

In addition to proper nutrition, you need to care for yourself. You'd be amazed how sore your body gets when you're lying down all day. The tricky part is figuring out how to deal with those aches and pains. For some of you, a bubble bath may be a great way to relax (as long as you have someone at home to help you in and out of the tub and you get the blessing of your medical provider). Remember to not make the water too hot and to avoid saunas and hot tubs. Even if you aren't allowed a bath, aromatherapy and special lotions can help you relax.

When it comes to finding ways to move your body, talk to your OB, doctor, or midwife about restrictions. You may be allowed to do gentle stretches or even a light prenatal yoga routine. What you are allowed to do to try and prevent blood clots or other issues depends on your personal situation. Remember, your restrictions will continue to change as your pregnancy progresses. Keep talking to your healthcare provider.

With my daughter, I was allowed to have weekly home visits from my chiropractor. Since she had been on bed rest with her third pregnancy, she knew how uncomfortable lying down all day could be and the associated aches and pains. After her clinic hours, she would come to my house and lightly adjust me on my couch.

In addition to her treatments, she provided great tips, as a mother who had been there. It was very helpful talking to a mom who had been on bed rest. She knew how isolating it could be, and made sure she had time to spend with me, never rushing. It was truly appreciated.

One week, when my aches and pains were particularly annoying, I decided to get a home massage. I looked up a mobile registered massage service online, admittedly from a massage therapy service I had never used before. Excited with my upcoming massage, I posted a comment about it on Facebook. As luck would have it my previous therapist, who had moved to another city, saw my post. Being trained as a doula, as well as a mother of four, she immediately called and quizzed me thoroughly — asking if I'd received permission from my OB (which I hadn't), as well as the qualifications of the massage therapist in relation to high-risk pregnancies (which I didn't know). She acknowledged while I may be in discomfort, I should cancel the massage. After all, I would feel horrible if I did anything to jeopardize my pregnancy. She assured me it would only be a few weeks until baby was born and I could go for a proper massage, without having to worry about complications. When I told this story to my OB, she confirmed I was not to have massages. She also made me cancel my weekly visits from my chiropractor as I got closer to my 36-week c-section date; it was good while it lasted.

It is important you find out what in-home services you are allowed. Remember, what was allowed in week one of your bed rest may not be allowed in week four. Always check with your OB or midwife first.

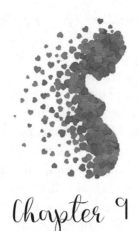

Chapter 9

Pack for the Hospital

There is no shortage of lists available on the Internet or in pregnancy books about what to bring to the hospital — for you and your baby. These are great lists to print to help guide you in packing your suitcase.

When you are on bed rest, it's important to have your suitcase packed and ready to go at a moment's notice. I had two bags; one for me and one for baby. When I had short-term hospitalizations for bleeding, I had my husband grab my bag, knowing I had time to bring the baby's bag later if needed.

It also helps simplify things for your support team to have your bags prepacked. A word of advice: Make sure it's clear whose bag is whose. In his panic, my husband one time accidently grabbed the baby's bag instead of my bag. Having a bag full of diapers and sleepers isn't particularly helpful when baby is still growing inside. After that incident, I kept my bag at the front door and left baby's bag inside of the crib (so there was no mistaking it was for baby).

In addition to the lists available on the Internet, here are some essentials to put in your hospital bag:

- **Granny cotton undies**. You know the kind — they go up to your belly button (which is a long way when you're pregnant). They are pretty much the most unflattering underwear you can buy. So why bring these crazy big undies? One word: c-section. Even if you aren't planning a c-section, when you're high risk the possibility is there. If you do end up with a c-section, your bikini underwear will sit directly on your fresh scar, digging in and reopening the scar. Trust me, granny undies will be your friend. Besides, there's no point ruining your good undies with what happens to your body after having a baby. I bought a supply of cheaper pregnancy underwear that could stretch to unnatural lengths and be discarded after baby was a few months old (that pregnancy belly tends to linger).

- **Healthy snacks**. This is a key component. Don't worry about packing candy and mints, as visitors will likely bring those for you. What they won't bring are some nuts, granola bars, crackers, or other guilt-free treats you may crave. Hospital food is lacking, at the best of times, and when you're pregnant or breastfeeding it can never fill your appetite. By packing some of your favorites ahead of time, you won't be filling up on the massive bag of jelly beans someone brought you. Make sure you pack enough to share; your partner will need some nourishment, too. Depending on how suddenly you are admitted, and the severity of your condition, your partner might not be able to step out and grab some food.

- **Books**. Any hospital stay before baby is born can get pretty boring. So make sure you have something to read. I had two emergency trips to the hospital where I did not pack a book. The magazine selection on the maternity floor was pathetic, and I was left reading breastfeeding pamphlets and four-year-old *People* magazines. Make sure you have a few books in your bag, as there is little to do while you're incubating. You might also want to throw in some magazines for some variety.

- **A long cardigan/sweater**. Leave the bathrobe at home. You'll want something to cover up or keep you warm but you won't want to be milling around in your bathrobe. Somehow wearing a sweater or cardigan feels less institutional and more like home. If your stay ends up lasting for more than a few days, you can have your bathrobe brought to the hospital for those early morning appointments. If you live a good drive from the hospital, then bring your bathrobe with you.

- **Charger for phone/iPad/laptop**. It's amazing how many people forget this crucial piece. Seriously, make sure you have this. It's worth buying a second one just to make sure you don't lose power on your device or it can make for a long day. Also test to make sure your backup charger works. I had thrown one in my bag only to discover when I got to the hospital it didn't work.

Exercise 5
Hospital Bag Checklist for Emergency Stays

This checklist will help you in packing your bag for the hospital. I'd strongly recommend having a bag with your items packed and at the front door in the event you need to head to the hospital quickly; see Exercise 7 for a packing list with more details. You can always have someone come and get baby's bag. Trust me, you do not want to have your partner or friend pack your bag for you once you've been admitted. Who knows what you will end up with?

Clothes
[　] Pants
[　] Underwear (normal and granny)
[　] Socks
[　] Nursing bra
[　] Comfy shirts
[　] Pajamas/nightgown
[　] Sweater/cardigan
[　] Slippers or slip-on shoes with good grip (not flip flops)

Personal items
[　] Shampoo and conditioner
[　] Soap
[　] Deodorant
[　] Brush
[　] Lip balm
[　] Hand lotion
[　] Compact mirror
[　] Hair elastics
[　] Panty liners
[　] Maxi pads
[　] Toothbrush
[　] Toothpaste

Sanity supplies
[　] Books
[　] Notepad and pen
[　] Nonperishable snacks (e.g., nuts, granola bars, dried fruit)
[　] Cell phone
[　] Laptop or tablet (check with the hospital about how to keep your valuables safe)
[　] Chargers
[　] Money (small amount)
[　] Blanket (that can get stained/dirty)
[　] Refillable water bottle
[　] Earplugs (in case you have a noisy roommate or to drown out hospital noises at night)

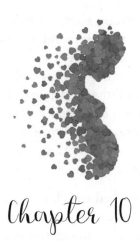

Chapter 10

Emotional Rollercoasters and Mental Health in Pregnancy

Being pregnant is a very emotional time for women. Add bed rest to the mix, and it can be a tearful experience.

Be prepared for all the emotions that come with being confined to the couch or bed on top of being pregnant. Having your independence taken away is challenging, and it can take a while to adjust. But remember it is only for a short period of time.

It's important to know you are not alone, even though there are many times you will feel you are the only person going through this experience. You may also feel that none of your friends and family understands or appreciates what you are going through. Despite these feelings, it may help you to know there are many other women feeling the same way right now, spending their days on bed rest. If you or a friend knows someone who has previously been on bed rest or is currently on bed rest, it is important to make the connection. Having someone to talk to who truly understands your experience and emotions can be a huge support. She can give you advice or just be there to listen, as she can relate to your experience.

If you don't know anyone, start searching online, looking for bed rest discussion forums. Ask your friends on social media if they know anyone who has been or is now on bed rest. Chances are you are only one or two degrees of separation away from making this important connection. Every few months, someone will ask me if I could talk to his or her friend who is on bed rest, or to give him or her advice, as a friend, on how to offer support. Once you have spent time on bed rest, you are part of a community of women, who are often more than willing to help a newcomer to the experience in any way possible.

During your time on bed rest, it's not uncommon to have moments when the stress and anxiety catches up to you and can be too much to handle. The smallest things can put you over the edge and cause a breakdown. And that's okay. We all have our breaking points, and having a good cry is actually therapeutic. It doesn't mean there's anything wrong with you or you can't handle the situation. It just means you're human and need to acknowledge your feelings and then let them go.

What set me over the edge in my confinement were airplanes going over the house; the Canadian Forces Snowbirds to be exact. For non-Canadians, the Snowbirds are an elite acrobatic team of pilots that perform at air shows across the country. They are incredible to watch and always draw large crowds.

I had read in the paper they were coming to town. Even though I'd seen them perform in the past, I was disappointed I wouldn't be able to go to the beach to watch them, as at this point in my pregnancy I was pretty much confined to the couch all day.

I was watching TV by myself and heard the planes fly over my house. Since I hadn't been off the couch for a couple of hours I went outside to sit on my deck to see if I could watch them. Unfortunately, the best view I could get was a one-second glimpse as they passed over the trees.

I went back onto the couch and broke down. I cried for at least half an hour. It wasn't about not seeing the air show, but rather the fact the choice to see the Snowbirds had been taken away from me. I cried for the loss of my independence. I cried for being alone while my husband was at work. I cried for all the stress and worry about my baby. This was the moment my bed rest caught up with me and I fell apart. For so long I had been trying to hold it all together. To put on a strong face for my friends and family and not admit I was scared and depressed. I had a good, ugly cry.

By the time my husband came home, I felt better. I decided to tell him about what had happened, as I was tired of putting on a brave face. It helped me realize that I wasn't OK and I needed to be honest about my feelings. We had a great talk about everything we were both going through, our fears, frustrations, and emotions. After that he was more aware of my emotions, and I of his. He reached out to some of my friends and family to let them know the struggles I was having, and asked them to check in on me — both with phone calls and visits. Through reaching out he learned that some people had been limiting their visits, thinking I needed to rest. Knowing that socialization was what I craved, they began popping by the house more often, for which I was grateful.

It's important our support team is aware of the emotional support we need. It can be hard to let them see beyond the mask, but now, more than ever, you need people to keep an eye on your emotional and mental health.

This is an area I found lacking in obstetric care. Your medical team monitors your blood sugar, blood pressure, baby's heartbeat, baby's positioning and more, but often the emotional state and mental health of mothers is overlooked. Too few medical providers take the time to talk with moms about the ups and downs of pregnancy and really find out how the mother is doing. Since no questions are asked, most women are reluctant to talk about their emotional struggles or feelings of depression, causing further feelings of isolation. It can become a vicious cycle with stress, depression, and anxiety causing pregnancy complications for both the mother and the baby. This is why it's so important to add the conversation about your mental health to your regular medical visits. After you've answered all the questions about your physical health, give your medical provider an update on how you are feeling, revisiting this throughout your pregnancy.

If you are struggling, make sure you talk to your medical support team or, at the very least, your partner or a friend. It's especially important if you've suffered from depression before you were pregnant or have a family history of depression. Even if you haven't, the raging hormones and isolation can impact your mental health.

You are at greater risk of suffering from depression and/or postpartum depression if you have one of the following risk factors:

- History of physical abuse

- History of sexual abuse

- Smoking during pregnancy

- Use of alcohol during pregnancy

- Use of nonprescription drugs during pregnancy

A 2014 Canadian Maternity Experiences Survey conducted by Health Canada found:

- 7.5% of women reported depressive symptoms postpartum

- 15.5% were diagnosed with depression or treated with antidepressants prior to pregnancy

- 12.5% of women reported that most days were very stressful in the 12 months before having a baby

- 13% had little or no support available to them during pregnancy

- Women who had been sexually or physically abused were highest represented in the above stats

If you are struggling or know someone who is struggling, there are some great resources in the Appendix.

I never shared my story with my OB, nor did she ever ask how I was doing emotionally. Nor did any of my friends or family as my brave face fooled them into thinking I was OK and taking the bed rest in stride. I was not.

Looking back I wish I had told my OB or family doctor, as I suffered from postpartum depression for the first few weeks after my daughter was born — also in silence. Thankfully by then I was blessed to have the supportive group of women that I met in my prenatal classes, some of who were also suffering and were open about their struggles. After our babies were born we met weekly, and sometimes multiple times a week. I also joined a second baby group through our local health unit. Two of the women in this group had also spent their last weeks of pregnancy on home-based bed rest. We were all having the same challenges recovering from months on the couch. It was these connections with other new moms and being honest about how I was feeling, that helped me through the early days of motherhood.

Jenn's Story

Jenn Mackey
Six weeks home-based bed rest
Mother of two

I was confined to bed rest early in my pregnancy due to preeclampsia or hypertension (high blood pressure). As a nurse, I knew how serious my condition was and the importance of resting. During my pregnancy I was careful about everything I put in my mouth, didn't drink caffeine, and did prenatal yoga. Despite doing everything right, I still ended up with complications.

The worst part of being at home on bed rest was being alone with my thoughts. I felt guilty about having somehow caused my condition. I was watching my body morph in size due to all the retained fluids and how sick I had become. It was very emotional for me to watch my body turn against me, as I'd always taken good care of myself. All of a sudden I had four chins and I didn't recognize myself. It was very depressing looking in the mirror.

What did help me during these difficult days was the routine I had established. My mother came for lunch every day, and brought me salmon sandwiches, as salmon helps reduce blood pressure.

I also set goals for myself. Some days my goal would be to take a shower. Another goal was watching the mini-series *Roots* as well as *North and South* before my daughter was born. Every night after my husband came home from work we'd sit down and watch one episode together. It gave us something to look forward to at the end of the day. It was a great distraction for both of us.

My cat also helped me get through the days. Due to all the extra fluid, I couldn't feel my baby move inside of me. My cat would lie on my stomach, and her ears would go up when baby moved. I would watch my cat to see my daughter's movements. This helped reassure me that she was still kicking away. However, I did feel cheated that I never felt my baby kicking.

Looking back on my bed rest, it was a surreal experience. At times I didn't feel worthy to have a baby, as my body struggled throughout the pregnancy. I experienced a lot of negative self-talk, and realize now that women need to be very strong to get through these emotions.

Having a healthcare background also helped me, as I was able to have real conversations with my medical team and get honest answers to my questions. I feel that many medical staff hold back information, not wanting to upset or scare patients.

The best gift I ever got from my OB was honesty. After a dramatic birth, with my daughter being born three months premature and my organs shutting down, I slowly began to recover. Once I started getting my strength back I told my OB I wanted to have other children. Through the relationship we had developed, he was honest with me. He told me if I were his wife he wouldn't want me to have more children due to the high risk of having even more complications during future pregnancies. This was tough advice to hear but it was the honesty my husband and I needed.

My biggest take-away from my bed rest and the time I spent in hospital after my daughter was born is how important it is to really talk about your feelings. Talk about your guilt, even when you have done nothing wrong, as it is a strong emotion that lives inside of you. If you don't, it will eat you alive.

Use a journal, talk to a friend, or confide in a member of your medical team. Do anything to work through your negative self-talk, anger, and guilt. You need to express these feelings, if only to yourself.

When you're faced with a crisis and are vulnerable as a patient, it is a difficult time. No one ever asked me how I was doing emotionally. Everything was about the baby. It would have been nice to be offered some help or talk to a social worker. I was offered support for breastfeeding, postpartum care, but never support for my mental health. I would have appreciated talking to someone about how my marriage was doing, financial pressures from not working, or my isolation from being on bed rest and then having a premature baby.

I encourage you to talk to your support system about all the challenges you are facing. All of these stresses can further complicate your pregnancy, your health, and your recovery. Don't wait until someone asks you how you are doing. Take the initiative to talk about your feelings and ask for the support you need.

I didn't say anything at the time, as I was afraid it would impact my care. But being a nurse, I now look back on my experience with a different perspective. My time on bed rest and having a daughter in the NICU changed my approach to my career. It has made me a better nurse and a better leader. I transitioned into management as I had lived the experience and had a fuller appreciation of the perspective of a patient. Our health care is so focused on the disease or complications, that too often the mental health aspect of how patients are coping is overlooked.

Don't let your personal needs be overlooked. As you count down the days until baby arrives, make sure you get the care and support you need so you are better prepared for the challenges coming your way as a new mom.

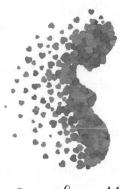

Chapter 11

Short-Term Hospital Stays

Some women on bed rest have the benefit of spending their bed rest days at home, with few complications, while others will pop in and out of hospital for short-term stays. Sometimes these short-term stays result in long-term admissions, which we will get to in Part 2 of the book, but for now I want to focus on short-term stays.

So what do I mean by short-term stays? At times the condition that put you on bed rest in the first place will require closer observation at your local or a regional hospital. This could be due to complications with gestational diabetes, high blood pressure, placental abnormalities, vaginal bleeding, leaking or low amniotic fluids, or preterm labor. Other times a hospitalization can be the result of factors unrelated to your original complication such as heat exhaustion, stomach flu, and dehydration. The lists of reasons for short-term hospitalizations are many, and admission is often unexpected.

As I mentioned earlier, my first hospitalization was the result of me overdoing it and breaking some rules. It was a hot summer long weekend and I really needed a new bra. I had to have it immediately. No debate. I convinced my husband to take me to the maternity store. After I found a bra that fit, I told my husband we might as well go out for supper, saying I had to eat right away. He had his doubts but I eventually broke him down. Being pregnant, I decided to go to the washroom before getting in the car and driving home. That's when I realized I was in trouble as I had quite a bit of vaginal bleeding. Enough to set me into panic mode and know I needed to get to the hospital immediately.

I got into the car and calmly told my husband to drive me to the community hospital where I had taken my prenatal class (which wasn't the nearest hospital). I called the maternity unit at the hospital on the way and, as luck would have it, the nurse teaching my prenatal class answered. Since she was well aware of my situation she told me she would contact the OB on call and would see me in five minutes (as we lived close to the hospital). When I told her I was 25 minutes away, she was confused. I then had to confess I had been out for supper and shopping. She said she would save the lecture until I got to the hospital and was admitted.

I was promptly admitted and given a stern lecture by the OB as I mentioned in Chapter 2. Yup, I definitely knew the rules after that lecture.

I would soon have company from another mom I knew who was admitted for a short-term stay. The next day, a nurse popped her head into my room and told me I had a visitor. One of the women from my prenatal class was in a wheelchair being pushed by her husband. The look on her face was pure terror. Even though she had a "normal" pregnancy, she had also overexerted herself in the heat of the long weekend and was being admitted for dehydration. She seemed relieved to see a familiar face, and when I told her why I had been admitted and my complications she calmed down, realizing her situation could be worse.

She spent the night being monitored and rehydrated and was discharged the following morning. When she left she gave me all of her magazines and a book, which was much appreciated, as the only reading material I had was a breastfeeding brochure that I had read about a hundred times — not the most exciting reading material.

We were both happy to see a familiar face on the maternity floor and know we were not alone. Her short stay also made me realize it wasn't just high-risk women who find themselves in the hospital. It even happens to women with "normal" pregnancies.

My next admission was the incident I mentioned where my real estate agent drove me to the hospital. That time, I was put in a semi-private room. For the first night I had the room to myself. However, the next morning a terrified young mom was wheeled in with her equally panicked husband. She was being admitted to monitor a placenta abruption (where the placenta tears away from the lining of the uterus). By now I was a pro at short-term stays (or so I thought). I put down the book I was reading (I was prepared this time) and struck up a conversation.

This was her first pregnancy, and up until now it was "normal." She was close to her delivery date, but still at the point that if her baby were born she would be preterm. I shared my story about my home-based bed rest, complications, and two hospital admissions, and she opened up about her fears and concerns.

We ended up bonding over our situations. The next morning her husband showed up with breakfast for both of us.

With both of these admissions, I was happy I was able to connect with other moms and was not alone. I was also glad I was able to share my experience with them as well as calm some of their fears.

However, in my excitement to be discharged, I lost track of the bigger picture and didn't advocate for myself. Both of my admissions had been the result of vaginal bleeding, which is a red flag (pardon the pun) for women with placenta previa as it could result in a massive bleed and preterm labor.

Looking back at the experience, and the lessons learned with my second case of placenta previa and a long-term hospitalization with my son, I should have asked to be transferred to a larger hospital to be admitted and where I would have been monitored closely throughout the remainder of my pregnancy (which is often the standard practice). Instead I let my desire to be home and put the hospitalization behind me outweigh the safety of both my baby and me.

When I shared these stories with the OB that looked after me during my pregnancy with my son, he told me the safest place for a woman with placenta previa in her third trimester (sometimes earlier) of pregnancy is in the hospital as a major bleed can happen suddenly.

I share this story so you can reflect on your own condition. If you feel uncomfortable about going home, or have more questions than answers, ask to be transferred to a larger hospital, even if it is a distance from your home. I was at a community hospital for my first pregnancy, that didn't see many high-risk pregnancies, as these were often dealt with at the larger hospital. However, there was a high-risk pregnancy unit (antenatal) less than an hour from my home that would have been better equipped to deal with my condition.

It is important that you be your own advocate. If you don't feel confident in this role, or have the energy, ask your partner, family member or friend to advocate on your behalf. Often, a short-term hospitalization is your body's way of telling you to pay attention. Sometimes it's just telling you to rest more, and other times it's saying it's time to get the care you need in a hospital setting — even if you'd rather be home on your couch. Don't worry, you'll spend enough time there once baby is born.

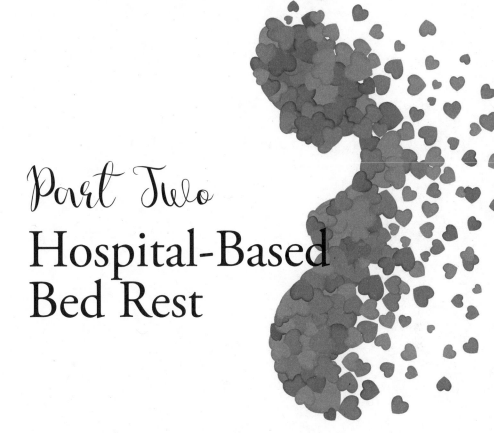

Part Two
Hospital-Based Bed Rest

While this section of the book is focused on hospital-based bed rest, at first glance you may notice what appears to be a duplication of text from Part 1 of this book on home-based bed rest. Just as there are some similarities between home and hospital-based bed rest, you will notice there is some repetition of information on various aspects of bed rest in terms of chapter headings and exercises. However, just as the realities of the two experiences differ greatly, so does the advice and guidance contained in the text.

I encourage you to read each chapter with fresh eyes, this time taking the perspective of a mom who is spending her bed rest in a hospital setting. Just as I advised at the beginning of Part 1, pay attention to the information that will help you in your particular situation and ignore the areas that are not relevant at this time. Remember, pregnancy, your restrictions, and your living situation can continually evolve and change, and you need to be open to this change.

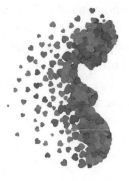

Chapter 12

Prepare and Pack
for Hospital

1. Prepare

It can be pretty daunting being told you're being admitted to hospital. It can be a sudden admission due to an emergency situation, a planned admission with a few days' notice to prepare, or an extension of a short-term stay into a long-term admission.

For women with high-risk pregnancies, the idea of a hospitalization often looms over them. In some ways this helps limit the element of surprise when you are finally hospitalized. In other ways it can add a level of stress to the pregnancy — knowing at any moment you may have to trade your couch or bed at home for a bed in the hospital.

However, women with high-risk pregnancies are not the only women who find themselves hospitalized during their pregnancy. As mentioned in Part 1 of this book, any pregnant woman can be hospitalized for a variety of reasons including stress, severe morning sickness, illness, anxiety, dehydration, or any other condition that puts the health of the mother or baby at risk.

In my six weeks on the antenatal unit (a unit for women being monitored during their pregnancies) I met dozens of women who were admitted for a variety of reasons. Some stayed for a couple of days, while others carried out the remainder of their pregnancy in the hospital. On my unit at a large teaching hospital more than an hour from my home, women were brought in from as far away as a 12-hour drive (many of these women were flown in by air ambulance). Some came with only the clothes on their backs, while others were given advance notice and had time to prepare for their admissions.

If you have advance notice of your hospitalization, there are some questions you'll want to ask to find out more about your stay (see Exercise 6). These will help you prepare emotionally as well as practically for your time in the hospital, and help you have a better understanding of your new environment.

2. Pack

Whether you have a few days to prepare or are asking a friend to pack for you after an emergency admission, this list will help you make your hospital room more comfortable and less institutional. Personalizing your room will help you get through the days, as you will be surrounded by familiar objects from home. Often, this personalization becomes a conversation starter with medical staff and fellow patients. I had a quilt on my bed that my grandmother had made with a mix of fabrics. I loved looking at it and all the pieces my grandmother, who had passed away many years earlier, had cut by hand. It made me feel like she was a part of my hospitalization and I wasn't alone. This quilt also started a number of conversations, with medical staff and patients asking about who made it and its history. I still remember some of the personal items that made each of my friends' rooms unique on antenatal, many looking less like hospital rooms and more like dorm rooms.

It's funny, the longer you stay, the homier your room becomes. I found my visitors would bring items to add to my space, such as a whiteboard for my wall, fresh-cut flowers from their gardens, or framed photos. By the time I was discharged after 43 days of living on antenatal, the entire trunk and backseat of our car was filled with

Exercise 6
Questions to Ask about Your Planned Hospital-Based Bed Rest

1. Am I going to be on an antenatal unit (devoted to high-risk pregnant women) or a maternity floor (mix of women high-risk, women in labor, and women with newborns)?

2. Will I be in a private room, semiprivate room, or ward?

3. Is it a large teaching hospital, regional hospital, or community hospital? If it is a teaching hospital, ask about the role of residents in my care, understanding the difference between visits from a resident (to get information about my condition) and visits from the OB or doctor (to assess this information).

4. What does my meal plan look like? Does it include snacks or only three meals a day?

5. How much variety is there in the menu? This is important for long-term stays. Some hospitals offer a separate menu for long-term patients to order from when they are tired of food on the main menu. Unfortunately these are usually unhealthy meals such as grilled cheese sandwiches, pizza, and burgers.

6. Does the hospital menu change often or does it repeat on a weekly basis?

7. How much does it cost for Internet, television, and phone? Is there a long-term plan available versus a daily rate?

8. Are there laundry facilities for patients to use? Where are they located? Is there a cost? Do I need to bring my own laundry soap?

9. Is there a television room or common room for patients? Where is it? Are there any restrictions to using this room?

10. If there isn't a common room, is there an opportunity for the women on the floor to get together?

11. Are there scheduled social activities for patients? Some antenatal units have daily programs in the common room.

12. Is there a place to lock up my valuables? This is important, as unfortunately theft in hospitals is a common occurrence.

13. Is there a refrigerator to store my food? Do I need to put my name on my food?

14. How much does parking cost? Can I buy a monthly parking pass for visitors to share?

15. What are the visiting hours? Can my child/spouse/friend spend the night?

16. Am I allowed to leave the hospital for short periods to go for dinner or coffee with a friend (or any short outing)?

Once you are admitted, your nurse will go over all these details with you. If you have a few days before a planned admission, it is good to get a tour of the unit as well as see a room, so you have an idea of what to expect and what to bring to the hospital. It helps relieve some of the stress if you can see in advance of your admission where you'll be staying.

---

items from my room. It took my husband multiple trips to load the car. When I looked back at my empty room, which now really looked like a hospital room, I was very grateful I had personalized the space to make it a warm and inviting room.

The following sections discuss some items you may want to bring to make your stay more comfortable.

2.1 Quilt/throw blanket

This will make your bed look less like a hospital bed as well as provide some needed warmth as hospital bedding is thin. This one item will provide the most comfort and personal touch for your room. Make sure it's machine washable and a blanket that can be stained. With IVs, blood draws and other tests, there's a good chance it will get stained. Also it should be made for a single bed, not double, to avoid the bedding getting caught up in the support rails of the bed or other equipment.

2.2 Pillow

Bring a comfortable pillow from home as hospital pillows are covered in plastic, which can make your head sweat, and are often as thin as a pancake. I recommend bringing a pregnancy body pillow like the Snoogle mentioned in Part One or another comfortable pillow from home. It may take up the entire bed, but it will make for a comfortable sleep. Be prepared for some staining due to the medical nature of being in a hospital.

2.3 Pictures from home

Decorate your room with pictures of family and friends. You may be spending a lot of hours staring at the walls, so make sure you have pictures that remind you of all the love and support you have for you and your baby. During my stay, I made some scrapbooking pages to decorate my walls (and I'm not a crafty person). I used ultrasound pictures (no shortage of those) to create a page for my son and had my husband print off pictures of my daughter to make a page for her. These were bright, colorful, and had positive messages on them. My daughter loved seeing her page when she arrived, and I like how it brightened the room. One friend brought me a corkboard where I was able to pin up pictures and cards.

2.4 Vision board material

When you're confined to a hospital bed it can be easy to get caught up in the medical tests and institutional feel, which can cause stress and depression. Creating a vision board will help you focus on the future you want for you, your baby, and your family. It helps take your mind off your hospital bed to focus on the future you want to create. Both the creation of the vision board and staring at it day after day will have a positive impact on your spirit and your surroundings.

A foam core board or poster board, scissors, old magazines, and tape are all you need to make your own vision board. Trust me, you'll have many hours to flip through magazines. You can ask your family and friends to give you their old magazines. Don't be picky as to what magazine, as you're just looking for words or pictures that are part of the future you want to create.

Simply cut out the pictures, words, and phrases that resonate with you. Once you have a supply of images that reflect your vision for the future, glue or tape them onto the foam core or poster board. Then prop this against a wall or window that is in your main field of vision. It serves as a visual reminder of the future that awaits you, your baby, and your family. You can add to this throughout your hospital stay, so you are continuing to work on your future. This will also become a conversation piece for visitors to your room.

2.5 Books

Reading material is always an important part of hospital stays. If you're staying in an antenatal unit, once you meet other women, you'll quickly be swapping books. You'll want a few to get you started. Reading a series, such as *Harry Potter* or *Divergent*, is a great way to pass the time. When I was hospitalized, the *The Hunger Games* trilogy traveled from room to room. Not only was it great sharing books, but it also gave us moms something to talk about. If you are admitted and don't have books, ask the nurses if there is a library in the hospital. There was a bookcase in my antenatal unit, but it was mostly filled with Harlequin romance books. However, I later discovered a parent quiet room on the pediatric unit that was filled with a variety of books, including many new releases.

2.6 Snacks

Whether or not the hospital provides snacks, trust me you'll want to bring your own as the hospital snacks can be repetitive. The snacks in my hospital were limited to prepackaged cheese and crackers, bananas, apples, and yogurt. While that may seem like a good selection, after a couple of weeks in hospital I was looking for some variety. Bring some nonperishable snacks for your room. Granola bars, nuts, crackers, trail mix, and a favorite treat such as popcorn or dark chocolate are good options. Don't pack too much candy or junk food, as your visitors will bring you more than you will want to eat. The common room is often full of junk food that discharged women leave behind.

Most patient kitchens have a kettle, but what they don't have are quality hot drink mixes. Don't even think about ordering a hot chocolate, tea, or coffee with your breakfast. By the time it gets to your room the water will be lukewarm. It's a good idea to stock up on some hot beverage mixes in your room. Even if you are confined to your bed, you will find a friendly hospital worker or visitor who will happily boil water for your drink. It's also a good idea to bring a mug from home, as the hospital mugs tend to be plastic and small. A thermal travel mug is ideal as getting up to warm up your drink could be a challenge.

2.7 Bathrobe, cardigan, slippers, granny underwear

You'll want something for a quick cover-up. A bathrobe is great for those surprise 7:00 a.m. ultrasound appointments, but you'll probably prefer a long cardigan when visitors come to see you so you don't look so institutionalized. As for slippers, make sure they are easy to get on and off and offer some support for your feet. Crocs are a great option as you can even wear them in the shower, which is important if you are sharing a shower with other patients.

Don't forget your granny underwear: I'm talking about the dreaded up-to-your-belly-button, super unattractive underwear. While it may look hideous, it is surprisingly comfortable. If you end up with a c-section, you are not going to want a bikini brief digging into your fresh scar. It's also a good idea to stock up on some granny underwear so you don't stretch or stain your good underwear. Remember that bit about how hospitals and pregnancies can stain your personal items.

2.8 Laptop/tablet/cell phone

In most hospitals, long-term television rental is expensive, whereas long-term unlimited Internet is affordable. Using FaceTime or Skype on your tablet or laptop is a great way to stay connected with friends and family without racking up minutes or data on your cell phone (unless you can find Wi-Fi for it, and download the Skype app to your phone). I used my iPad every night to read bedtime stories to my daughter. I had some of her books in my room. I held them up to the iPad every night while I read the story. It was a great way for me to be a part of her bedtime routine and it also gave my husband a break as I entertained her — which was needed for him, with me being in a hospital 1.5 hours away from home.

2.9 Money

You will want some cash so you can go get a coffee or visit the gift shop. Make sure you have your bank card in case you need more, as most hospitals have an ATM. Always lock up your money when you're not in your room. This is important for all of your valuables, as theft in hospitals is sadly a common occurrence. During my stay, food and personal items went missing from patient rooms on a regular basis, particularly rooms that were out of view of the nurses' station.

Exercise 7
Hospital Bag Checklist for Your Preplanned Hospital Stay

This checklist will help you in packing your bag for the hospital.

Clothes
[   ]   Pants
[   ]   Underwear (normal and granny)
[   ]   Socks
[   ]   Nursing bra
[   ]   Comfy shirts — long and short sleeve
[   ]   Pajamas/nightgown
[   ]   Sweater/cardigan
[   ]   Slippers or slip-on shoes with good grip (not flip flops)
[   ]   Housecoat

Exercise 7 — Continued

Personal items

[　] Shampoo and conditioner
[　] Soap (hand soap and shower soap)
[　] Hairbrush
[　] Lip balm
[　] Hand lotion
[　] Face lotion
[　] Deodorant
[　] Razor
[　] Compact mirror
[　] Hair elastics
[　] Panty liners
[　] Maxi pads
[　] Toothbrush
[　] Toothpaste

Sanity supplies

[　] Books
[　] Notepad and pen
[　] DVDs
[　] Nonperishable snacks (e.g., nuts, granola bars, dried fruit)
[　] Cellphone
[　] Laptop or tablet (check with the hospital about how to keep your valuables safe)
[　] Chargers
[　] Money (small amount)
[　] Blanket (that can get stained/dirty)
[　] Refillable water bottle
[　] Earplugs (in case you have a noisy roommate or to drown out hospital noises at night)
[　] Nursing bra
[　] Comfy shirts – long sleeved and short sleeved

Comfort items

[　] Blanket
[　] Pillow
[　] Pictures from home
[　] Books and toys (for visits and online calls)

Items for the long haul

[　] Nursing pads
[　] Earplugs or noise-canceling headphones
[　] Eye mask
[　] Bath towel(s) and wash cloth(s) – the ones in the hospital are rough and small
[　] Nonperishable snacks (e.g., nuts, granola bars, dried fruit, chocolate)
[　] Hot drink mixes (e.g., hot chocolate, tea, coffee)
[　] Mug and/or travel mug
[　] Refillable water bottle
[　] Phone, charger, tablet
[　] Money
[　] Vision board tools (e.g., scissors, tape, glue stick, foam core, or poster board)

Lisa's Story

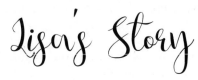

Lisa Gow
Nine weeks hospital-based bed rest
Mother of two

This is the story of my nine weeks in hospital while pregnant with my twins. I hope by sharing some of the tips I've learned it will help you during your stay.

At 27 weeks of pregnancy a routine visit to the local hospital for my biweekly ultrasound showed a shortened cervix. I was instructed to carefully go home, pack a bag and be driven three hours to the regional hospital specializing in neonatal care. My husband and I arrived at the hospital tired, scared, and reeling.

The intake nurses were calm throughout my tests, blood work, and getting me settled. Everyone seemed to have done this so many times that it was old hat and they didn't consider all the questions that a first hospitalization would have let alone a first-time mom. Once in my room the real fear set in.

Doctors and genetic specialists swamped us with information. While it was all delivered with the best of intentions, the tone was accusatory. As if I wanted to have my babies so early that they would have major development issues!

We were scared speechless. We couldn't form intelligent questions. So we bumbled along for a few weeks until I got a feel for the establishment and found my groove.

Here are some tips from my 63 days of being institutionalized.

1. Bring a great chair into your room. Bed rest doesn't always mean staying in bed. It does mean relaxing with your feet up — so a zero gravity chair is your new best friend. The hospital visitor chairs are seriously uncomfortable for long periods. So if you want company (you do) ask for two chairs for your room.

2. There are volunteers and staff that will wheelchair you outside for fresh air. ASK. Ask frequently. Get outside.

3. There are restaurants and cafeterias you can be taken to for a change in diet. Many local restaurants will deliver to the nurses' station. Keep some cash and order in some of your meals. Not plastic. You'll need cash if you are sharing a delivery order with other moms. Also ask the hospital about alternate menus. We had access to the special menu for the children's ward. After 30 days even Kraft Dinner looks very appealing. If you see a menu item you like, order multiple meals in the morning and save them for a time when the meal of the day doesn't appeal to you. Ask to use the kitchen fridge or the staff room fridge. You will need Ziploc bags and masking tape for labels. A sharpie is handy too.

4. Ask for physiotherapy. Muscle atrophy is going to be a problem and any exercise you can do that is doctor approved is going to benefit you when you are finally released.

5. Early morning wake ups can be avoided. Be awesome to the residents the first few weeks and they might just overlook your room on the weekly rotation. The breakfast tray can also be delayed at the door if you choose.

6. Laundry. You need detergent and coins. I was very lucky to have a cousin come in twice a week to remove and return my clothes. She was a Godsend.

7. Keep a journal. Not so much else to do and it does all fade away. I enjoy looking back at the stages of success from my time in the big house.

8. Make friends. People will come and go as their conditions change, but meet and greet as much as you can. Why watch

TV in your room if you can go to a common room? It makes the time go faster, lightens your mood and if you are very lucky, some of the friends you meet may turn out to be life-long ones.

My twins were born hale and hearty at 36 weeks 6 days at my home hospital on their originally scheduled c-section date. Thanks to the nurses, doctors, PT team, Cousin Jill, and friends that visited (some with ice cream) as well as the antenatal mommas. You're the best!

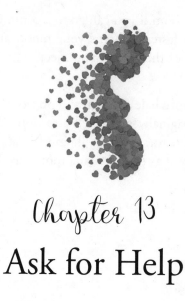

Chapter 13

Ask for Help

Once word gets out you've not only been put on bed rest but also admitted to hospital, you will have friends, family, and neighbors saying to you and your partner "let me know if there is anything I can do to help." You'll likely brush away these offers, saying you're fine. After all, they're just saying that to be polite. Right? Wrong.

Don't guess others' intentions. By accepting support and asking for help you'll soon find out who is sincere. And this is a time when you truly need that help. But before you ask for help be clear on what it is you need. Here's a list of some areas you might need help while you're in the hospital, unable to do your normal things.

Support at home:

- Rides for your children
- Caring for your children
- Meals for your family
- House cleaning
- Laundry

- Grocery shopping

- Setting up baby's nursery

- Shopping for baby's arrival

- Picking up relatives at the airport

- Setting up your baby registry

Support at hospital:

- Visiting you

- Snacks and home cooked meals for you

- Driving your children to come visit

- Doing your personal laundry

- Bringing supplies to hospital

- Taking you out (if allowed this could be a quick trip to a restaurant or outdoor space)

Asking for help can feel awkward. It's tough to know who is sincere about their offers and who isn't. Here's a tip I used when I was put on home-based bed rest with my daughter and again when I learned I was being admitted to hospital while pregnant with my son. I sent an email to friends, family, and coworkers providing an update on my pregnancy. Since I had been placed on bed rest with no warning, I never had a chance to say goodbye to my coworkers or let friends know of my hospitalization in advance.

In the email I clearly listed how my husband, daughter, and I needed help. This was less awkward for us as I wasn't directly asking anyone for help, so no one felt obligated. In the email I stated the help we needed and let people decide if and how they could help.

I knew, in my absence, my husband wouldn't reach out and ask for help but would definitely appreciate any support he could get, particularly with our daughter.

The response was overwhelming and help came from the most unlikely places. A cousin who lived 45 minutes from the hospital made weekly trips to keep me company, often bringing treats for me to share with some of my new friends in antenatal. A friend and former coworker visited me in hospital twice a week, bringing her small son with her. They soon became a part of our antenatal group, hanging out in the common room with our group of big bellies. This friend also took me out for small outings, including spending Mother's Day enjoying a seafood feast at a restaurant near the hospital. A close high school friend who lived a short drive from the hospital picked me up every week, took me to her house and, not only made me supper, but also washed my laundry. This was greatly appreciated as the washing machine on my floor was broken for most of my time in antenatal.

Back at home, a mom I had met at my daughter's dance class, who had spent part of her first pregnancy on hospital bed rest, took my daughter to her dance classes. She knew exactly what I was going through, and knew the best way to help was to take some of the load off my husband in caring for our daughter. Another mom bought flowers for my husband to give to my daughter after her dance recital — knowing he would likely forget. And the list went on.

Not only was I grateful for the support we received, but it also strengthened old friendships and created new friendships. I was beyond impressed with the willingness of friends, and near strangers, in taking time out of their busy lives to help my family during this challenging time. They took an active role in my pregnancy, and when my son and I were finally discharged from hospital, continued to help me as it took time to recover from my bed rest and c-section.

You may want to find your own way to ask — but make sure you do ask for help and are clear on your needs. By asking for specific help, your support network can help you in the way that works best for them. If you don't ask for help, not only are you adding unnecessary burden to yourself and your partner, but you also deny yourself the opportunity to let people in and support you in a way that works for them. You may also miss out on some amazing experiences and connections that come from lowering your defenses and asking for help.

Of all the exercises in the book, Exercise 8 can be the hardest for many women: Asking for help. For this reason, I want to push you out of your comfort zone and have you spend time being clear on what help you truly need and how your friends/family can best support you and your family.

My hope is by doing this exercise you take time to really reflect on your current situation and your personal and family's needs. When you've completed the exercise, please share this information with your family and friends who want to support you but don't know how or are waiting for an invitation from you.

Now take some time to answer the questions in Exercise 8. Remember, you may be asking for help from people who don't know you as well as your close family and friends.

The final task is to ask for help in a clear and specific way. How you do this can vary on your relationships. You can send a mass email to all of your friends/family/coworkers using the template or have individual conversations using this exercise as a tool on what your specific needs are, both now and after baby is born. What is important is that you are specific on the support you need and your family needs and how each person can help, filling in the chart as people respond. This chart should then be put on your fridge at home, with another copy in your hospital room. This way you can work with your partner or support at home to ensure they are accessing all the help available. It will also help you know who to thank when you are finally settled at home with baby.

Exercise 8
Asking for Help from Family and Friends when in Hospital

How long will you be in the hospital? Until baby is delivered or until your condition stabilizes?

How long do you expect to stay in hospital after baby is born? Are you having a c-section? Is it anticipated the baby will need extra care (NICU)? Will you need extra support?

How many children do you have at home? Ages?

What are your limitations after baby is born in caring for your children?

What activities are your children involved in which require support? Examples: tutoring, sports, clubs, school. Be specific on times, dates, locations.

Who typically prepares the meals in your family?

How are meals currently being prepared for your family?

What types of meals does your family enjoy?

If friends were to provide food, what is the best way of helping you in meal preparation?

Example: Prepared meals that just require heating or preportioned and chopped ingredients for a family member to put together. Be clear on what foods your family likes so you don't end up with a freezer full of tuna casserole no one will eat.

What support does your family need inside of the home?
[   ]   Cleaning
[   ]   Laundry
[   ]   Meal preparation
[   ]   Organizing baby's room
[   ]   Shopping
[   ]   Other _____

For the children
[   ]   Homework support

[   ]   Play dates or babysitting
[   ]   Lunch preparation
[   ]   Shuttling to activities
[   ]   Driving them to see you in the hospital
[   ]   Getting on/off the bus (be specific on times and pick up/drop off locations)
[   ]   Bath care
[   ]   Bedtime
[   ]   Other _____

What friends/family/coworkers have offered support (the "let me know if you need anything" statement)? Also include anyone would could provide support both locally and remote.

What are your greatest stresses?

How many days/weeks do you have until your due date?

Now review the questions and, in a different color pen, answer the same questions based on your anticipated needs after baby is born. Remember: Women who have been on bed rest often have a harder time "bouncing back" versus women who have been mobile throughout their pregnancy. This can be due to muscle atrophy and other pregnancy complications. A c-section versus vaginal delivery will require more time for your body to recover.

The next step is to review your answers and fill out the following chart. The column on the left is support needed. In the row on the top fill in the names of friends and family members who can help, checking the appropriate support they can provide based on your relationship and comfort level. I've left room for other forms of support.

SUPPORT NEEDED							
Inside the home							
Meal prep							
Cleaning							
Organizing baby's room							
Laundry							
Shopping							
Groceries							

Exercise 8 — Continued

For the children							
Homework support							
Rides to activities							
Play dates or babysitting							
Lunch preparation							
Driving them to visit you							
Getting on/off the bus							
Bath care							
Bedtime							

This table will help you visualize how the people in your life can help you in a variety of ways. It will also help you break down the support you and your family needs into specific areas and tasks, which will then show you where your friends and family can best offer their support.

Example 2
Draft Email to Family and Friends when in Hospital

Hi family and friends,

I'm sorry for this group email, but I've found this is the best way to communicate and provide an update on my pregnancy. As some of you know, I've been admitted to hospital for the health of my baby and myself. This is a stressful time for my family as I'm no longer able to be at home.

Some of you have offered your help. Instead of putting anyone on the spot, I thought it would be best to send a group email letting you know what support I need so you can let us know if you're able to help in any way.

What I need help with includes:
[edit this list to suit your needs]

In the home

- Laundry
- Cleaning
- Meal preparation (either helping at meal time or supplying healthy prepared meals) *[Be specific here on what you and your family like and don't like. Does this include making school lunches, snacks, meals?]*
- Organizing baby's room
- Grocery shopping

For the children

- Homework support
- Play dates or babysitting
- Bath care
- Bedtime

Outside the home

- Drop off/pick up of children from school/daycare *[be specific on times/locations]*
- Shuttling children to extracurricular activities *[be specific on dates/times/locations]*
- Driving kids to see you in the hospital

I'm hoping this list will help you better understand the support our family needs both when I'm in hospital and when I return home. My family and I are happy for any help you can give.

I also welcome any visitors to see me in the hospital. Before you visit, please send me an email or text so I can let you know if I have any appointments so I don't miss your visit. Also, I may need your help in bringing items to the hospital for me so advance notice of visits is appreciated.

I will continue to update you on this journey and thank you for all your love and support.

[Your name]

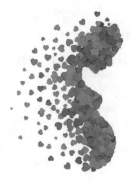

Chapter 14

The Early Days of Hospital-Based Bed Rest

The first few days of living in the hospital are the hardest. This is the time when all the residents, doctors, and support team come to visit you. While they are required to tell you the worst-case scenarios about your situation, it can be pretty intimidating. I remember being shocked with the amount of information coming my way. One doctor recognized this and apologized by saying "unfortunately in medicine we need to tell you the worst that could happen. Imagine if your car recited your chances of being in an accident or being killed every time you started the engine. You'd never drive. But we are required to tell you the worst case every time we speak to you."

This calmed me a little bit — until the next doctor came into my room. What helped me most was talking to another mother on my unit who had similar conditions as me; suspected placenta acreta (placenta attached to an organ, not the lining of the uterus) and complete placenta previa (placenta covering the cervix). Since we were admitted at the same time, we received visits from the same medical team on the same days. This was pretty convenient for everyone involved, including us two moms.

Although we came from different backgrounds, she was Amish and almost 20 years younger than me, our shared experience helped us connect as mothers. After visits from our medical team, we'd compare notes, talk about what freaked us out, and ask each other questions. This helped both of us dissect information and deal with stressful news, as we knew we were not alone.

I also became her go-between, asking her uncomfortable questions to our medical team and relaying the answers back to her. Since most of the doctors were male, she didn't feel comfortable asking questions about a potential hysterectomy or sex after a c-section. I had no problem getting personal. She began to open up and trust me through these conversations, and, in turn, began joining the other moms in the common room for our daytime conversations, whereas previously she had spent most of her days in her room. She became part of our long-term-stay group of friends, friendships that were formed over our shared bed-rest experience.

Over time, I found many mothers with similar conditions opening up and sharing notes in the common room. We were very candid about our conditions and what we were going through. When meeting new patients, we would always ask them why they were there. Then moms with similar conditions would welcome them and fill them in on what tests they could expect and anything they might want to know about their condition. This helped form friendships and connections, and alleviate some of the fears of new patients while building our little community.

Until that community is formed, if it ever is, it can be lonely sitting in your room — especially if you have other children at home. My first day at the hospital, I cried for an hour after my husband left. I cried every time I heard my daughter's voice on FaceTime. I cried when she came to visit and had to leave. I cried when other children came to visit their moms while my daughter was at home. I cried more than I ever had in my life. And that's OK. It is to be expected that you will miss your family. After all, living in a hospital is tough at the best of times. However, worrying about the health of your baby makes incubating even more stressful.

If you are staying at a hospital with a Neonatal Intensive Care Unit (NICU), early on someone will likely visit you from the NICU to talk about what happens if your baby is born early. Let's face it: High-risk moms are prime candidates for having babies in the NICU. I was offered a tour of the NICU, and I took it out of nosiness. I thought it would be my only chance of seeing a real NICU, as I did not think my baby would spend time there. I was 31-weeks pregnant, and the nurse showed me a 31-week-old baby. That was a wake-up call. I had no idea how small a baby is at 31 weeks. The baby websites and comparisons to different fruits didn't prepare me for the true size of the baby growing in my belly. It was good motivation for me to follow my OB's orders.

After my son was born I was very grateful for taking the opportunity to tour the NICU early in my admission, as he went into respiratory distress minutes after birth and ended up spending 13 days in the NICU. During my tour, the nurse clearly explained how the unit worked, the nurse to baby ratio (which depends on their medical issues), showed me some babies, and introduced me to the medical team. If I hadn't have taken this tour I would have been worried about where my son had been taken when he was born as it was hours before I was able to see him due to my own post-operation complications. Thanks to the tour, I knew he was in great hands and could even visualize his room. This allowed me to relax and focus on recovering from my general anesthetic.

Welcome these opportunities to ask questions of the medical team, tour the NICU, and learn what you can about your birth plan that your medical team is developing (which is much different than a low-risk pregnancy birth plan which is often created by the mother). Also, if allowed, venture out of your room to the common room on your floor. It can be very isolating spending your days alone in your room. However, great friendships can be formed with other women who are living under similar conditions.

During my stay on antenatal, our group bonded over food. In my first week, I helped organize a pizza party in the common room. Another mom and I went room-to-room inviting moms to the supper. We had ten moms join us for pizza. Some of these moms had not previously left their rooms or talked to other patients. Many were isolated and feeling very alone, staying hours away from their homes. The first pizza night, which evolved into a weekly tradition of avoiding Salisbury steak, started some amazing friendships that continue today.

Although we all came from different backgrounds and communities and were a wide range of ages, we bonded over our shared experiences. We even tallied up all the different complications we had amongst us, with placenta previa being the most prevalent condition followed by shortened cervixes and then leaking or low levels of amniotic fluids. We always joked about what team we belonged to, proudly stating our conditions.

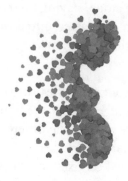

Chapter 15

Hospital Schedules and Early Mornings

It's worth having a discussion upon admission about when you will be woken for tests and doctors' rounds. This will help you determine what schedules are preset and the ones that are variable.

Adding to the sleep challenges of being pregnant, are the nurses, doctors, cleaners, and other hospital staff that will parade in and out of your room at all hours of the day and night. While you can try and sleep through some of these visitors (like the middle of the night nurse visits to check your vital signs), other visits will be harder to nap through.

One morning while I was in hospital a nurse came into my room at 6:00 a.m. to put a container for a urine sample on my bedside table. Not being a morning person and frustrated by yet another sleep interruption, I sat up and asked her why she was doing this at 6:00 a.m. (and not in the friendliest way). Her response: because it's Tuesday (urine day) and she was told to make sure all patients had their urine sample containers. I then told her she had an entire 12-hour shift to distribute the containers and us moms had the entire day to pee in them. I explained how hard it is to get sleep in a hospital, and she should wait until the women were awake before distributing to any more moms.

She sheepishly apologized and left my room saying she was only following orders. She did stop distributing the containers, waiting instead until the breakfast trays were delivered.

After I had properly woken up (as there was no getting back to sleep after this encounter) I asked to speak to the charge nurse (head nurse). I explained to her what an average day looked like for us patients, with all the medical visits and tests, and how challenging it was to sleep in a hospital with all the bells ringing and other noises. I painted the picture of hospital life from a patient's perspective before talking about the needless distribution of urine sample containers when women were sleeping instead of waiting two hours until the breakfast trays were distributed, which would wake the women. I took the time to let her know how the nurse's task was waking women unnecessarily, adding an additional stress.

By advocating for not only myself, but also the other women on the unit, the nurses changed their routine. For the remainder of my stay they waited until breakfast was served to come into patients' rooms. This was a change I, and the other moms, were grateful for.

I found in my stay that many times the hospital routine is set with little regard to the patients and their needs. This was also true with cleaners coming into rooms while moms were napping. If they went about their work quietly it wouldn't be an issue. But rather they would sing to themselves or try to have a conversation, not caring the patient in the bed was trying to sleep. While this is frustrating, if you take the time to explain your concerns to the charge nurse or someone else in authority, a compromise can be made. When it came to the napping, I would put a sign on my door saying Patient Sleeping — Do Not Enter. I would tell my nurse I was taking a nap for one hour, and would ask for some quiet time. For the most part, this request was respected. But I had to have the conversation in advance, versus expecting hospital staff to understand a napping mom wants to be left alone.

When it comes to doctors' rounds, you won't have much say in their schedules. Once again, it's good to be prepared. I was at a teaching hospital, where the residents did the morning rounds (anywhere between 6:00-8:00 a.m.) and the high-risk OB team did afternoon or early evening rounds. The residents, whom we got to know very well as they were on one-month rotations, made an effort to start their rounds as late as possible (closer to breakfast time). If they needed to have early rounds, they would often tell us the day before and let us know they would keep the conversation quick, asking us to let them know if we were having any medical challenges. Otherwise, they would check our vitals and leave.

It may take a bit of time to develop the relationships with the medical staff to set your boundaries. However, it is important they see you as a person, not a patient. This can only be done by having honest conversations with your medical team and getting to know them as people too.

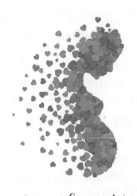

Chapter 16

Dealing with Mom Guilt

Being admitted to hospital for an extended period of time when you're pregnant is a unique situation. In many cases you are not sick, but rather being monitored or lying in bed to prevent an early delivery. This is different from many of the other patients who often have short hospital stays and are recovering from a procedure, surgery, or illness.

Not being sick, but spending days and weeks in a hospital can be isolating — particularly if you have children at home. Compounding this isolation is the fact that antenatal units are usually only located in large hospitals, meaning many women need to be hours away from their families and friends. If you are in a community hospital, you will likely be staying on the maternity floor. This means you will be surrounded by women in labor and the sounds of crying babies, which isn't ideal when you're trying not to have a baby.

Now add the layer of "mom guilt": The fact you are lying in a hospital bed unable to care for your child or children at home. Of all the pressures weighing on a woman on bed rest, I have found the stress of being away from children to be of greatest concern to moms. In my group of friends on antenatal this was a common conversation piece, with many women breaking down in tears on more than one occasion over missing their children.

There was one mom on my unit that rarely interacted with the other moms. One day when we came into the common room after breakfast we found her sitting on the couch crying. She had been talking to her son on the phone and he had been upset, begging her to come home. Her son was only three years old and didn't understand why mommy was so far away and he couldn't see her. This mother had been airlifted to the hospital from a community that was a ten-hour drive away. She had come in the middle of the night with only the clothes she was wearing. When she had gone to her local community hospital with complications, she had no idea it would be three months before she would see her son and be home again.

The stress of her middle-of-the-night admission, the great distance from her family and friends, and the bed rest restrictions put on her was too much for her to handle. She was set on going home and seeing her son, even though the medical team had told her this would put her baby's life at risk. She was so caught up in the guilt of being away from her son, that all she could think about was seeing him again.

A couple of the moms from my unit sat with her, letting her cry. We then explained that we were all moms who had left our children at home, and were feeling the same mom guilt. But we were also moms to the babies growing in our bellies, and at this time, the babies in our bellies needed their moms to care for them. We needed to focus our attention on these babies; doing everything we could to help keep them safe, just like our partners or family members were at home keeping our other children safe.

After an hour of crying and other moms sharing their fears, concerns, and stories, the mother calmed down. She realized she wasn't alone and that the women around her were going through the same challenges. It also helped her to be reminded that the baby in her belly was her child too and needed her full support and attention.

While this might all make sense to you, it doesn't mean there won't be moments where you break down, missing your child or children. For some of you, this might be the first time you've been away from your children for more than a few nights. In addition to your sadness, your children are likely also suffering from their own separation issues.

When I was in the hospital I was concerned my absence would somehow scar my three-and-a-half-year-old daughter. I was afraid she would feel that I had abandoned her or didn't care about her. When she would cry, asking me to come home, my heart would break. At times I thought I was a horrible mom, not being able to be at home to care for her.

Here's what I learned: Yes, my daughter missed me and wanted me to come home. But she also loved her extra time with her grandparents and the one-on-one attention she was getting from her dad. Young children live in the moment. The here and now. When they are talking to you, they want you, but when they are at daycare or school, their attention is focused on what they are doing.

It is like when you drop your child off at daycare. He may cry and scream, but often will settle down by the time you are in your car, happily playing with friends. He wants you when you are there, but when you are gone, his attention refocuses to what is in front of him.

This is often the same way with being away from your child while in the hospital. It doesn't mean she won't miss you or that you shouldn't talk to her for fear of upsetting her. Rather, that children process information much differently than adults.

I also found it is important to share with your children's caregivers what is going on with your pregnancy. I made sure my daughter's daycare was aware of our situation, so they were prepared for any behavioral issues or changes.

Now that it has been a few years since my hospitalization, when I talk to my daughter about the time her brother was in my belly and I was away from home, she has very little memory of it. She remembers the ice cream she ate in my room, playing in the indoor playground on the pediatric unit, and pushing me in a wheelchair. She doesn't remember any of the crying or have a concept of how long I was away from home.

Looking back, it's a bit of a blur for me too. However, in the moment, it was at times all-consuming. When I was finally discharged,

I made sure I set aside one-on-one time with my daughter, even if it was to read a book with her cuddled in my lap while her brother was sleeping. I cherished every minute, as did she.

1. Connecting with Your Children at Home

There are a number of ways you can stay connected to your children at home, and provide some relief to family or friends who are caring for your children.

1.1 Skype/FaceTime

Set up a time each day to connect with everyone at home. Make sure this time works for your medical support so you won't be interrupted for tests or doctors' visits. I found 7:00 p.m. was ideal as it was shift change for the nurses (so they were busy), the day's medical tests were complete, and my daughter was getting ready for bed. The daytime nurse would let the nighttime nurse know I was talking to my daughter, and would like privacy until 8:00 p.m. By having a set time each night, my husband was able to set a timer for my daughter so she knew when she could call, and the nurses knew when to leave me alone. It gave us both something to look forward to during the day. Some nights the nurses would come into my room while I was talking to my daughter. They would check baby's heartbeat, letting her hear her brother inside of me. She loved being a part of this nighttime routine, and it made it real to her that I had a baby inside of me. This is why I needed to be in the hospital, away from her.

1.2 Establish a routine

Beyond setting a time for daily calls, there are other things you can make a routine out of for you and your child(ren) to look forward to. For us, it was bedtime stories.

Since my daughter was young, I had a stack of her picture books in my hospital room. I turned the iPad camera to her books and read her bedtime stories every night during our chats. While I read the books, my husband would either clean up the kitchen (while my daughter was at the kitchen table) or would take the time to rest himself. If you have school-aged children, it might be a good time to help with their homework via phone or computer. By reading her bedtime stories I was able to be a part of her nightly routine, even though I wasn't there in person. It allowed me to stay connected to her.

1.3 Set dates for a visit

If it is possible, have your family set dates for visits. Knowing in advance when you will next see your children gives you something to look forward to while you are apart. If you have young children, you can also help them understand when you will see them. Count down the number of sleeps, mark it on a calendar in their room, or talk about what you will do when they come (read books, eat ice cream, go for a walk). The hospital I was at had a children's playground in the pediatric unit. Antenatal moms were allowed to bring their children to this playground during visits. It was the highlight of my visits with my daughter as it was much more fun than sitting in a hospital room — for both of us. I was able to watch her just being a kid, playing with toys, or doing crafts, while my husband and I got caught up.

1.4 Special connections

I had one of my daughter's stuffed animals in my hospital room, on the window ledge next to my bed. When we would FaceTime I would show her the toy and create a story about what the toy and I had done during the day. She loved knowing her toy was on this adventure with me. It also comforted her to know I wasn't alone, but had her toy watching over me. The nurses would sometimes examine her toy after they had checked on her brother's heartbeat. They would put a bandage on the toy, saying they were looking after the toy and her mom.

When my daughter came to visit she would take the toy home and give me a new toy. Deciding what toy to bring was also a conversation piece in the days leading up to her visit, with her showing me the different toys in her room, trying to decide which one needed to go spend time with Mommy.

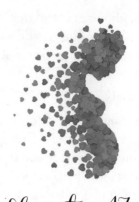

Chapter 17

Rainbow Babies

I didn't learn the term "rainbow baby" until I was hospitalized with my son and the moms on my unit were sharing stories of previous pregnancies. A rainbow baby is a baby conceived following a miscarriage or infant loss. Both of my children are rainbow babies.

The majority of the women on my floor were carrying rainbow babies, having lost babies anywhere from 6 to 39 weeks during their last pregnancy. Many of these women were no strangers to high-risk pregnancies. For some it was their previous loss or high-risk pregnancy that put them in the antenatal unit, so they and their babies could be closely monitored. For others it was a recurring pregnancy-related condition (preeclampsia, shortened cervix, leaking or low amniotic fluids, problems with the placenta) that put them at earlier risk of preterm labor or threatened the health of their babies.

Regardless of their conditions, moms carrying rainbow babies also carry with them an added layer of stress and anxiety. We are the moms who know all too well that with the joys of pregnancy could also come great sadness and loss. While we were excited and optimistic about the babies growing inside of us, we were always cautious and a bit fearful that something could happen to end the pregnancies.

Once we discovered we were not alone, and shared our previous losses, we were able to talk openly about our fears and anxieties. We also had a better appreciation for what each woman was going through, and how best to provide support.

If you have not experienced a miscarriage or infant loss, I don't share this piece to scare you, but rather to help you understand some of the emotions of moms who have had a loss. A mom who may appear standoffish or quiet, may be doing her best to cope with her hospitalization while still grieving a lost child. The hospital may also bring back unpleasant memories, and for some, they may be staying in the same hospital where they had their pregnancy loss.

For the moms reading this book who are carrying a rainbow baby, please remember each pregnancy is different, even if you have a recurring pregnancy condition. I have known moms who have suffered great loss yet defied the odds and have a healthy, albeit preterm baby who is now a busy school-aged child. While infant loss is sadly always a possibility, so is the possibility of having a healthy baby. Know that you are exactly where you need to be in case there are any additional complications in your pregnancy. The hospital is indeed the safest place for you and your baby.

Nicole's Story

Nicole Bontaine
Eight weeks of hospital-based bed rest
Mother of three

The pregnancy that landed me in hospital on bed rest was a pregnancy that was a few years in the making. My husband and I had tried to get pregnant naturally, with oral drugs and two attempts at intrauterine insemination (IUI) — no luck.

On Halloween we were accepted as foster parents for an 11-month-old girl, with the expectation we would eventually adopt her (which sadly didn't happen). Four days later we were scheduled for our third round of IUI. We decided to go ahead with the procedure as we were financially invested and the adoption was not guaranteed.

While we were adjusting to being foster parents, we found out we were pregnant with triplets.

I was sent to the larger regional hospital for weekly ultrasounds as I was considered a high-risk due to my age (37) and the fact I was carrying three babies.

When I was four months pregnant I fell on the sidewalk, rolling my ankle. The doctor said it did not affect my pregnancy, but part of me will always feel this accident is what caused my son to get sick. A few days after this accident, I was told he wasn't growing at the same rate as the other two babies.

At five months pregnant, I was admitted to hospital as my son's condition was diagnosed as reverse blood flow in the umbilical cord, which was limiting his development. The OB explained it was too early to deliver the babies, as his sisters weren't strong enough yet to leave the womb. The plan was for me to hold out until 30 weeks when I could get a steroid shot and deliver all three.

My husband and I prayed on the decision and decided to wait.

I had daily ultrasounds and was closely monitored. I was able to hear their heartbeats every day and feel them move.

On the night of May 16, all three babies were moving great. The next morning the ultrasound technician couldn't find a heartbeat for my son. I was one day shy of 30 weeks and the steroid shot. My son Nolan had passed away. Miraculously I didn't deliver my triplets until 33 weeks, 4 days, giving my daughters time to develop.

Every perfect gift comes from God above. We were blessed with triplets to cherish and love. Born together, to grow apart, two daughters in our hands and one son in our hearts.

What I was feeling

I remember being afraid all of the time. Sometimes, it was easier not to think about it, but it didn't mean I wasn't afraid. I was afraid of falling. I was afraid I was alienating people. I was afraid of not gaining enough weight. I was afraid for my husband, feeling guilty for having him handle everything at home. Mostly I was afraid of exactly what happened … going to that one ultrasound to hear those words, there is no heartbeat. But being afraid didn't stop it from happening.

I was also sad a lot. I was missing out on our foster daughter at home, on my parents' arrival to help us, on my friends, on my life; it all made me sad.

Despite this sadness, I have to admit I liked the time to rest and not having to do housework with a bulging belly. I looked full term at five months, so it was difficult to do almost anything.

I also liked having meals brought to me and taken away. The antenatal ward felt like you were catered to: Whatever you wanted, when you wanted it!

I did expect people to come visit me. It helped the time pass. These visits made me closer to some family and friends, and created some distance with others who did not come to visit. I now know how it feels to be hospitalized and the important role visitors play.

Making friends

The best thing about my experience was the friendships I created while in hospital.

The first week of my admission, a very happy lady came to my room to see if I wanted to be part of a pizza night in the lounge. Am I ever glad I did. Becoming friends with the ladies around me helped immensely. It helped to have someone to talk to, who didn't know you so you could tell them what you were truly feeling and not worry about being judged.

It took away the loneliness, the sadness and helped with the fears.

It helped the day after losing my son. When my husband left [for the day], this virtual stranger whom I met a month ago, sat with me in my room, and held my hand while I cried. She didn't shy away from me. She didn't let me curl up in a ball and succumb to the sadness and pain that was ripping me apart. She checked on me daily until I was ready to come out of my room and be a part of life again.

These ladies would play games and go to the meetings and courses offered by the hospital. They would talk, they would listen, and they were my rocks while in the hospital. To this day they are the people I turn to for advice, and to share my concerns.

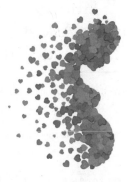

Chapter 18

Know the Rules:
Types of Hospital-Based
Bed Rest

When you're first admitted, your OB or nurse will likely run through the rules of your stay. This often involves going through your treatment plan, leave of absence opportunities, as well as restrictions. During this conversation make sure you are clear on your restrictions so you know what to expect during your hospital stay, recognizing your restrictions will likely change as you get closer to your due date.

The following are some questions to ask about bed rest and other aspects of your stay, in Exercise 9. If you have been admitted without notice, also refer back to the preadmission questions in Exercise 6.

Exercise 9
Questions to Ask about Your
Hospital-Based Bed Rest

Do I need to stay in my room all day? If not, for how long can I leave my room?

May I go to the common room? Is there a limit for how long I can spend in there sitting up?

May I walk to the common room or do I need to go in a wheelchair?

May I go for a walk in the hospital? If so, how far? (Be specific on this one.) May I go to the coffee shop on the first floor or to the cafeteria on the other side of the hospital?

May I go for a tour of the hospital in a wheelchair? (Always good to have a change of scenery.)

May I go sit out front of the hospital? In a wheelchair or can I walk?

May I get leave of absences to go for supper outside of the hospital with a friend? If so, how far away from the hospital am I allowed to go? For how long?

Am I on a special diet or can I eat what I like?

What warning signs should I watch for?

How often will I see an OB? How often or will I see my regular OB?

What are the visiting hours?

Can I have a visitor sleep overnight? My child?

Can I take my own medications (including naturopathic) or just those prescribed?

Exercise 9 — Continued

Is there a place to lock up my valuables?

Can I tour the NICU?

Can my visitors bring me flowers or balloons (some hospitals have restrictions)?

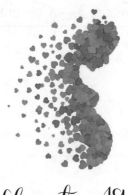

Chapter 19

What Tests to Expect when on Hospital-Based Bed Rest

If you are admitted to hospital, you are there due to concerns about the health of you and/or your baby. This means nurses, residents, OBs, and possibly even other types of specialists will closely monitor you. In addition to visits from your medical team, this monitoring could include tests such as ultrasounds, non-stress tests (NST), urine dips, weigh-ins, blood tests, and more.

The following sections offer brief descriptions of some of the tests you might encounter during your stay. You will have lots of time in the hospital to ask your medical team to better describe your care plan and the tests involved for you as an individual. The descriptions are just a quick overview of what you might expect.

I highly recommend highlighting the tests you have questions about and sitting down with your doctor or nurse to discuss each test as it relates to your personal care plan.

1. Ultrasound

The frequency and complexity of ultrasounds (also called sonograms) depends on your condition and can vary throughout your pregnancy. There are two common ultrasounds: fetal growth and condition-specific. A fetal growth ultrasound is one tool for your medical team to check in on your baby. It measures four areas: movement (body or limb movements), breathing (baby taking practice breaths), tone (extension of leg/arm and/or opening and closing of hand), and amniotic fluid volume. If the baby fails in any of these areas (which can happen to even healthy babies when they don't feel like cooperating), you could be sent for a non-stress test (NST) to ensure baby is OK and not in distress. How often you have one of these ultrasounds depends on your condition. For mothers expecting multiples, or extremely high-risk situations, it can be as often as once a day.

The second ultrasound focuses more on you and your condition. This could involve measuring amniotic fluid volume (too much or too little), baby's positioning, placenta positioning, placenta abrasion, and more. Once again, the frequency depends on your condition and how far along you are in your pregnancy.

The ultrasounds will be conducted at your bedside (for extremely high-risk or ill mothers) or in medical imaging areas at your hospital.

2. Non-Stress Test (NST)

For this test you will lie on a bed while equipment is strapped to your belly to measure baby's heartbeat and movements. Each time you feel the baby move you click a button. This is measured against the movements captured by the monitor. It also helps pass the time and gives you something to focus on during the test. The monitor will capture baby's heartbeat to record its average rate, as well as any accelerations or decelerations (which is normal). The fun part of this test is hearing baby's heartbeat and seeing the movements on a graph.

3. Urine Dips

At a minimum, you will be required to provide weekly urine samples. These are to monitor your sugar levels (to watch for gestational diabetes) as well as check for pregnancy-induced high blood pressure (preeclampsia). Depending on your condition, you may have more frequent urine tests. Thankfully, it is usually not a problem getting a pregnant woman to pee.

4. Blood Draws

The frequency and reason for blood tests also varies based on your condition. Blood draws are part of the routine for women with placenta previa to cross-match blood in the event a blood transfusion is needed (due to a massive bleed). It's a proactive test to prepare the medical team in case the worst happens. For women with gestational diabetes, sugar levels may be tested several times a day with a simple finger prick.

5. Weigh-ins

For some women, this is the most dreaded test of all, but it shouldn't be the case. After all, putting on weight is a normal part of growing a baby. Concerns arise when a mother gains too little or too much weight, which can require further investigation. Don't get hung up on the number on the scale, as long as you are approaching your pregnancy in a healthy manner. The nurses on my floor told us to look away and they'd quietly write down the number, as it was just for their records.

6. Medical Team Visits

Be prepared for multiple visits from medical and support staff, especially during the early days of your stay. If you are in a teaching hospital, this will also include visits from residents, increasing the amount of people stopping by your bedside.

While some people resent the visits, I enjoyed the new company. I became friends with some of the residents. After all, I saw them daily for a month until they switched rotations. A few came to visit me after my son was born as they had a genuine interest in our outcome.

Preparing for daily medical visits is key. On antenatal units, a team of high-risk OBs rotate the daily rounds, often with one OB on rounds for a week at a time. In anticipation of their visit, I would write out any questions I had, including asking for permission to leave the hospital for a short supper with a friend. These leaves of absence are reviewed on a daily basis and are dependent on your current situation and medical examination.

During the weeks my OB was on rotation, I had a lengthy list of questions. He often left my visit to the end of rounds, knowing I would want to talk. He even wrote "socialize" on my chart, recognizing how important it was for me to connect with him. Thankfully we had a great relationship and our talks helped ease my fears of my upcoming c-section, which had a few anticipated complications. By the time the c-section date arrived, and I learned I would have a general anesthetic so I wouldn't be awake for the birth of my son; I was fine with the decision as I had full confidence in my OB. I also fully understood the course of action, which was to keep my baby and me safe.

This confidence came from my talks with my OB during his rounds. I also had confidence in and respect for the other OBs on the team, as I knew they saw me as a person, not just a patient, which was important to me.

Take the opportunity during rounds to ask questions and, more importantly, to get to know your medical team. Also, be engaged in your birth plan. My birth plan was complex and took weeks to fully develop. However, being involved in discussions each step of the way helped me understand what was to come.

Social workers, physical therapists, dieticians, and spiritual counselors may also visit you. Once again, take time to engage in conversations with these people on your team. They can offer support as well as become friendly faces during your stay.

In talking to the spiritual counselor, we discovered we were from the same hometown and shared stories that took my mind away from the hospital. In a conversation with the social worker, I offered advice on what items the hospital foundation could fundraise for to help women in antenatal. After my son was admitted to NICU, many members of my support team visited his incubator while I was recovering from my surgery. It meant so much knowing he was hearing familiar voices when I wasn't able to be with him.

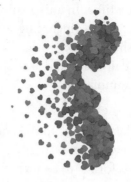

Chapter 20

What the Heck Is a Birth Plan?

A birth plan for high-risk women is much different than one for our low-risk counterparts. It's less about what type of music you want playing as you breathe through contractions and more about feeling you have some input into one of the most important days of your life. Even if your birth plan isn't followed (which is also often the case for low-risk pregnancies), it will help open conversations with your medical team about your thoughts, fears, and wishes. It will also help you feel you have some sort of input into the birth of your child.

While there are many birth plan templates available on the Internet, they are more appropriate for low-risk pregnancies. These templates are a starting point for those of you who are anticipating having a vaginal delivery. They cover the basics, including:

- Pain control usage preference for mom during labor (e.g., Demerol, epidural)

- Labor and delivery positions

- Assisted delivery preference, if needed (use of forceps or vacuum)

- Delivery of placenta (natural or assisted)

- Mood of the room (music, noise level, who is present)

However, I would caution that due to the simple fact you are on bed rest and have a high-risk pregnancy, you are less likely to have control over the items listed above. If you are having a c-section (scheduled or emergency), many of these items will not apply to your delivery.

When I was on antenatal while pregnant with my son, my OB spent a few weeks developing my birth plan. Since the medical team had originally thought I had placenta accreta (placenta growing through the uterus and attaching to an organ), my OB needed to consult with a number of specialists to work out the details of my c-section. My birth plan was a medical guide of various scenarios; tests needed prior to my c-section; a summary of specialists involved in my case; as well as potential worst-case scenarios and related courses of action.

While the best case scenario was a planned c-section where all the appropriate medical staff were in the room (which thankfully was what happened), my OB needed to be prepared for an emergency c-section, especially if he was not in the hospital and an OB unfamiliar with my complicated case needed to do the surgery.

As more information about my case became available, thanks to the numerous tests I had, the thick binder that contained my birth plan was updated. The goal was to have a summary of the most current information and course of action in the event I went into labor.

While the majority of my birth plan was created by my OB, I still had the opportunity to review the plan and provide my input. However, in talking to other moms, I have learned that this opportunity is not always offered. So don't wait for your OB or medical team to sit down with you and ask you what input you want into your birth plan. Rather, ask them to review the plan with you so you understand what they have planned for your delivery. Make sure your thoughts and needs are also included in the plan, recognizing they may or may not be followed depending what happens at the time of delivery.

In my case I was able to have the information in the following exercise contained in my birth plan because I had a good relationship with my OB and I had had a previous c-section with delivery complications. For my first c-section I was completely unprepared for baby being whisked away from me at birth (she needed medical attention) and being too weak to hold her in the first few hours (due to heavy blood loss). Thankfully my husband stepped up to the plate, and fulfilled my desire to have skin-to-skin contact in the first few hours, and delayed the use of formula until I was able to breastfeed.

Looking back, I wished I had written down my thoughts, so my husband and the medical staff would have known my wishes when I was unable to speak for myself.

For my son's delivery, I learned the night before the c-section that I would be having a general anesthetic not a spinal, as my OB and I had discussed. The anesthesiologist strongly felt it was the safer option due to my complications. Thankfully I had not only discussed my postdelivery wishes with my OB and husband, but also had them included in my medical birth plan.

When my son was born and rushed to the NICU, and I was still in surgery, my husband was able to be my voice. For the first few days, until I got my strength back and was able to clearly communicate my wishes, my husband referred to the birth plan on areas such as feeding my son formula until my milk came in, hand expressing my colostrum for my son's feeding tube when he was too weak to nurse and providing skin-to-skin contact with my son.

Developing your birth plan will not only help your team know your wishes, it will also help you work through the various scenarios related to delivery and postdelivery, so you feel better prepared.

Exercise 10 will help moms with high-risk pregnancies and deliveries work with their medical teams in creating personalized birth plans.

Exercise 10
Develop Your Birth Plan

Fill in what you can on your own, and then sit down with your OB or medical provider to go over what you've written and help fill in the gaps. This could start an important conversation and ensure you are both on the same page when it comes to your delivery day. Once your birth plan is complete, ask for copies to be made. Have one copy inserted into your medical chart, give your partner a copy, and keep one copy for yourself. This way, where possible, your desires will be followed even if you are unable to speak for yourself.

Anticipated delivery method

[   ]   C-section

[   ]   Vaginal

[   ]   Vaginal birth after a c-section (VBAC)

Who do you want in the delivery or operating room with you?

Who can make decisions on baby's care if you are unable?

Who can make decisions on your care if you are unable to speak for yourself?

How far into pregnancy do you expect to delivery your baby?

[   ]   Term – 37 weeks on

[   ]   Late preterm – between 34 and 36 weeks

[   ]   Moderately preterm – between 32 and 34 weeks

[   ]   Very preterm – less than 32 weeks

[   ]   Extremely preterm – at or before 25 weeks

If possible, do you want to hold your baby after delivery?

If possible, after delivery do you want to do skin-to-skin contact (with baby lying on your bare chest)?

If you are unable to do skin-to-skin and your baby is not in the NICU, do you want your husband, partner, or family member to do skin-to-skin with baby? Who?

How would you like your baby to be fed?

[   ]   Breastfeeding

[   ]   Breast milk (possibly a donor's)

[   ]   Formula

If your baby is in NICU and you are unable to nurse, do you consent to formula being used until your milk comes in?

Do you want a consultation with a lactation nurse after baby is born?

If your baby is in NICU, who do you consent doing skin-to-skin holding with the baby in your absence?

If your baby needs to be transferred to another hospital who should go with him or her? Is this person authorized to make decisions regarding the baby's care?

If it is a boy, do you want him to be circumcised?

If yes, in the hospital or at a later date?

Do you have a name for the baby?

Is there anyone who is not allowed to visit baby?

Is there anyone who is not allowed to visit you?

How soon after having your baby do you want visitors? (Some women prefer waiting 12-24 hours to give them time to rest and to bond with baby.)

Other questions:

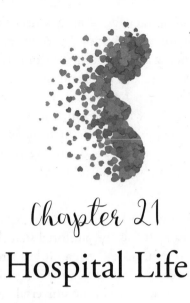

Chapter 21

Hospital Life

Whether you're in an antenatal unit, on a maternity floor, or in a regular room, hospital life can be an eye opener. Everyone around you is there because they are ill, are in labor, or their baby is at risk. While there are many happy endings and a few miracle babies, unfortunately not all outcomes are good.

There is no preparing for hospital life. Some of it is exciting, such as hearing a mother in labor then hearing her baby's first cry; other events can be traumatic, such as hearing a code blue (cardiac or respiratory distress) being called over the PA system.

I debated if I should include this section in the book, but I thought it would be a disservice not to as I was completely unprepared for the complexities of hospital life when I first entered the hospital.

Hospital life is loud. There are monitors beeping, patients buzzing for the nurse, conversations in hallways, and announcements on the intercom. While you do get used to this noise after awhile, it is still disruptive. That's why I recommend packing earplugs or noise-canceling headphones. They will come in handy.

There are other hospital codes you may hear that can be disturbing, including those for a missing or aggressive patient. A few times during my stay a code white was called (aggressive patient) and the nurses closed the doors to our unit and our individual room doors until the incident had been resolved. This was especially disturbing when I was in the NICU with my son, and I assumed the momma bear pose, standing behind the door in front of his incubator. I'm not sure how much of a threat I would have been with my post c-section, hunched-over body, but I was determined to protect my son, if needed.

When I was admitted to hospital no one explained the codes to me, or what they meant. It was the janitorial staff that helped me understand the codes, which made them a bit less stressful as they were shouted over the intercom. I'd recommending Googling what the codes means for your area, as there is no universal set of hospital codes.

In addition to codes being called, medical issues can happen at any time. My first night in antenatal, the woman in the room next to me gave birth at 28 weeks. The nurses closed my room door, but I could still hear all the commotion. It was a scary introduction, but the nurses reminded me that's why we were in the hospital; so we could get immediate medical attention if needed.

Partway through my stay, a group of moms were sitting in the lounge watching TV, when one mom got up to go to her room — and did not return. She wasn't feeling well, so she went to her room and called the nurse who immediately contacted the OB. She had heavy vaginal bleeding from her placenta previa, had gone into premature labor and needed an emergency c-section. Her son was born at 32 weeks and admitted to NICU, where she stayed at his bedside for many weeks, in a bit of a daze.

Her sudden departure, mid-TV show, was a scary moment for all of us, making us realize anything could happen at a moment's notice. It also made us appreciate the constant monitoring and support we were receiving. Had she been at home, the bleeding would have been a life-threatening event. Thankfully, she was staying on the antenatal unit, only a few feet from the c-section operating rooms.

Once her son had stabilized, she came back to antenatal for visits, watched TV, and took much needed breaks with us. She told us how much she valued having the opportunity to chat with other moms who had been with her through the hard part of her pregnancy. We each took turns visiting her baby, which also helped us become more familiar with the NICU and its staff.

When my son was admitted, this mother and her son were two incubators down from us. It was reassuring to have an NICU veteran help me in the early days. She showed me where to get the breast pumps, how to sterilize the equipment, and where to get clothes for my son. It was also great to have a friend to grab a coffee with between breast pumping sessions.

While hospital life can be unpredictable it can also be rewarding. One mother of twins found out she was going to have a c-section, even though she had planned for a vaginal birth. She was clearly terrified at the idea, and was shaking when I saw her in the hallway.

Having had one c-section and scheduled for a second, I went to her room and told her about my experience. Her OB had explained the medical side, but I was able to give her the mom's perspective. I walked her through my experience, from getting gowned up and prepared in my room to being taken into the operating room without my husband, to the having the spinal block (pain medication inserted into the spinal fluid for c-sections to "freeze" the lower half of the body) and then the actual procedure as well as recovery. My detailed explanation of what I went through, as well as my emotions, helped calm her. It didn't take away her fears, but it helped her have a better understanding of what was to come. After a few minutes of talking she stopped shaking, and gave me a big hug. I was glad my experience was able to help another mom.

You also need to find "normal" moments, a few minutes a day where you do something from your normal, non-hospital life. For me, it was drinking coffee. When I was pregnant with my daughter I followed all of the rules, not eating sushi, soft cheeses, luncheon meats, or drinking coffee. For my son I followed most of the rules, but allowed myself a few cups of coffee a week. After all, for most of my pregnancy I had a preschooler to look after.

In the hospital I stayed at there was a café the floor below the antenatal unit. I discovered it early in my stay, and got permission from my OB to take the elevator, walk the few feet to the café, and order a coffee. I would then take the coffee to my room, close the door, and read a book. For the 30 minutes it took me to drink the coffee and read my book, I felt normal. It was my zen moment. I did this three times a week, right after breakfast, before the unit got too busy with activity.

Find your zen moment. It could be picking up the phone and chatting with a girlfriend or watching a favorite movie or even painting your fingernails. The idea is to set aside a few minutes, with the door closed, to do what you would do in your normal life. It will help get you through some of the not-so-normal moments.

As mentioned in Chapter 14, you should also talk to your medical team about leaves of absence. Depending on your condition and current situation, you may be able to have a friend or family member take you out of hospital for a short escape. The rules of your outing will be clearly defined for you (how long you can stand/sit/drive, and when you need to be back in hospital). I had one friend take me shopping to a store that had wheelchairs. For a glorious 30 minutes I was wheeled through the store, and was able to pick up some baby items for my son, school supplies for my daughter, and some decorations for my hospital room. I also had outings for supper, a trip to the farmers' market, and visits to a friend's house. These outings, which were usually limited to two hours, did wonders to boost my mental health and make me feel like a normal pregnant mom, if only for a few minutes.

1. Privacy

One aspect of the numerous exams a mom on hospital-based bed rest goes through is the amount of people coming in contact with your body. If you are uncomfortable with others seeing you not fully clothed, it might be time to get over your inhibitions. Or find a way to keep your dignity while being examined (wearing tops and pants versus dresses). If you are a particularly modest person, my advice is to remember every test and exam is in the best interest of you and your baby. As mothers we will do anything for our children. Just think of your hospital stay as the first step in a lifetime of putting the health and safety of your child first, even if it means exposing your belly to a room full of strangers. If you're fortunate enough to have a vaginal delivery, there is much more show and tell yet to come.

Nicole's Words of Wisdom

Nicole Bontaine
Eight weeks of hospital-based bed rest
Mother of three

Here is some advice from lessons learned during my eight weeks in the hospital. I hope this advice will help you during your stay.

1. Make friends with other people in the hospital if you can. Don't let age differences, religious differences, social status, any other differences hold you back. Make the effort to talk to the people around you. You will be pleasantly surprised by what you actually have in common.

2. Be nice to the staff. They will be nicer to you and someone you can talk to. Everyone has a story and sometimes it was nice hearing about the custodian and her granddaughter, a movie the person giving you the ultrasound had seen, or a story from the porter pushing you to ultrasound. They all have lives, and sometimes talking to them can be a lifeline to the outside world.

3. Be kind, even when you are having a bad day. Realize that some of the comments you make can be hurtful, and you won't always get a chance to see that person again to say sorry. I think about the ultrasound technician who discovered my son Nolan's heart stopped beating and had to get the OB to confirm this. In my grief, I was not nice to her. Luckily I did get the chance to apologize after I was readmitted. But had I not been readmitted I may have never seen her again and would have felt guilty about not apologizing.

4. Pray. Have something to believe in: God, Buddha, Allah, whatever makes you get through the days. Don't underestimate the power of prayer and belief in getting you through what can be a lonely time.

5. Read, watch Netflix, plan, and organize. Knit, crochet, draw — do all the things you wanted to do but never had time. Once your child comes, it will be a long time before you can — so take advantage of the time now.

6. Expect your friends and family to help and be there for you and your family at home. But don't be mad if they don't help in the way you expect. Sometimes people are limited in what and how they can give. Appreciate any help and accept it graciously.

7. Don't let self pity and wallowing take over your existence. It is very easy to fall into the woe is me world. Make the best of the situation even if it hurts to smile. Recovery is harder when you let yourself fall deeper into depression and anxiety.

8. If you experience a loss, give yourself time to grieve. Allow yourself to carry reminders of the life that was lost. I have a tattoo on my arm that signifies the hardest day of my life, when my son's heart stopped beating. When I look at it, it is a reminder that no matter how bad or hard today is, I have had a harder day, and survived.

I have a teddy bear with Nolan's ashes in it and we included this in all our family pictures. I also have a necklace with his ashes that I wear when I need him close to me. Each year, on May 17, I allow myself to feel everything: The pain, hurt, anger, injustice, peace, hopes, anticipation of seeing him one day; everything I want to feel on this sacred day without any guilt.

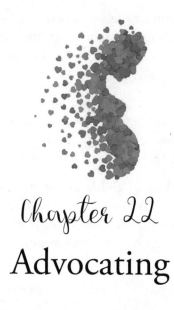

Chapter 22

Advocating

I've touched on the importance of advocating for yourself earlier in this book, but want to revisit this subject for the moms who are in hospital. Even though you are a patient who is being cared for by a variety of medical staff, it doesn't mean oversights won't happen. You still need to be aware of your medical condition, any changes in your body, and advocate for yourself.

While I found the vast majority of medical professionals were kind, dedicated, and attentive, like any profession there were some individuals who should have chosen a different career. The first time I was sent for a non-stress test (NST), the nurse hooked me up, gave me the fetal count clicker, and told me to hit the button every time baby kicked. That was the extent of the instructions. She then left the room. I had no idea how long this test was to last. About an hour later another nurse stuck her head in the NST room, and was shocked to see me lying there. It turns out the first nurse had forgotten about me. I also learned it was common practice for nurses to stay with the patient throughout the 20-minute test, which was something the first nurse had not done.

A few weeks later I had the same nurse again. Part of the protocol for women with placenta previa is to have blood drawn every three days, to be cross-matched in case a blood transfusion is needed. Since I had gone through this regime for two pregnancies, I knew the routine and kept track of the days between blood draws.

In the morning, I asked my nurse when she would be drawing my blood. She brushed me off saying she was busy. I asked her again in the afternoon. No response. The night shift was also too busy to take my blood.

I was unlucky enough to have this same nurse three days in a row and asked again the next day, but still no blood draw. On the third day of having this nurse, I told her to stop what she was doing and to listen to me. I told her that the blood draw was an important part of my care, and she needed to take the time to take my blood. She mumbled to herself, left the room and returned with my chart. Upon entering my room, she said, "Well, you can quit your nagging. You were right. You do need your blood drawn." After she had taken my blood, I asked to see the charge nurse and complained about this nurse. It turned out other moms on the unit also had challenges with her, and the nurse had told them she did not like working antenatal, as we were too demanding. We were all happy when she was reassigned to the maternity floor.

While I really did not enjoy being a pincushion with regular blood draws, I knew it was an important procedure in case I had a heavy bleed. After that, I kept even closer track of all of my regular appointments, such as ultrasounds and NST, and a few times during my stay I had to remind the nurses when I was due for these tests.

I was not the only mom to experience challenges. We soon learned which nurses were there to support the patients and which nurses would rather be working elsewhere in the hospital. We had one nurse who was the mother hen of our unit. We would all wait until she was working to ask our personal questions or share our concerns. She truly cared about the emotional and physical well being of the women on the unit.

During your stay, try to make a connection with at least one nurse, so you have someone to talk to about your concerns. This nurse can also help you navigate less supportive medical staff, especially if you are not comfortable advocating for yourself.

Jen's Story

Jen van der Meulen
Seven weeks hospital-based bed rest
Mother of three

At around 20 weeks into my pregnancy I was diagnosed with a low lying placenta and was due for additional follow up ultrasounds to make sure my placenta was moving in the right direction; away from my cervix.

At 29 weeks I started spotting. I was taken for further testing. My placenta was low lying but didn't seem to be an issue. Because my spotting stopped while I was in hospital I was sent home.

A few days later, I woke up to more blood and back to the hospital I went. At this point the ultrasonographer was mad because she was busy and I had just checked out and now they were sending me to be checked again. She once again declared I was fine.

The doctor decided to send me to a larger teaching hospital for follow-up tests. I was told to have my husband pack an overnight bag for us as I may have to stay there one night. I wasn't allowed to drive home.

I got to the teaching hospital and the resident came to talk to me about my placenta previa. I told her I had never been diagnosed with that and had no idea what she was talking about. She seemed shocked no one had warned me about this condition and she was certain I had it. She also let me know the devastating news that I would not be leaving the hospital until the baby was born at least seven weeks from then.

I got admitted to my room in antenatal and spent the first night crying. There was so much going through my head. What if this pregnancy ended badly like the previous two? What about all the stuff I had to do before the baby arrived? We still hadn't picked up the crib and the room wasn't ready. I always told myself my baby's room would be ready a month before I was due, being as so many of my friends had gone three weeks early. What about the farm? We run a dairy farm. I was an essential part of everyday operations so I had to find relief help.

I was going to be stuck in the hospital alone as my husband had to go back and run the farm. I just couldn't believe this was happening. A few hours prior I didn't even know anything was wrong with me. I had this guilt that I couldn't even just have a "normal pregnancy."

The following day I went for a follow-up ultrasound, with an internal ultrasound. They discovered that I did in fact have placenta previa. I had been misdiagnosed. I had an extra lobe on my placenta that was hanging down over my cervix, and due to the angle could only be seen with the internal ultrasound. Through the weeks I was in hospital, I had several episodes of bleeding, blood taken every three days, non-stress tests, ultrasounds, etc.

For the first two weeks I didn't leave my room very much. I tried to go out to the social activities in the lounge but not many other women were there. Sometimes I went to watch TV in the common room or check my email but no one else ever seemed to be around. I mostly went out of my room to just have tests done.

About two weeks into my stay, two other women staying in antenatal came into my room wondering if I wanted to avoid another Salisbury steak Wednesday, and we could order a pizza instead. I was hesitant at first; after all, shouldn't I just stay in my depressed little bubble? However, Wednesday's hospital meal really was the worst and I made the choice to join them, and that was the best decision I ever made.

There were about eight of us who decided to do the meal together, and it was the start of some amazing friendships. To this day (five years later) a group of us still get together several times a year and we always celebrate the babies' birthdays together. Those who choose not to come out, or are unable due to distance, are still connected on social media.

Now I am thankful for how it all turned out. Had I not been sent to a teaching hospital in London, and had I gone into labor naturally in a local hospital where there wasn't always an anesthesiologist on staff, this pregnancy could have been fatal for both the baby and me. I also wouldn't have met this wonderful network of friends!

My greatest advice is having some source of entertainment. Mine was watching the *Gilmore Girls* seasons on a portable DVD player, reading, puzzling, and being social. Don't let depression get the best of you. There is always something better to look forward to.

The key is if you are stuck in the hospital on bed rest, there are likely other women in there just like you, yearning not to be alone. You are all in the same situation, allow that to bond you and not divide you.

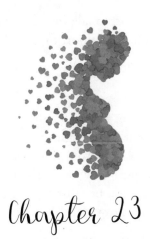

Chapter 23

Socialization

1. Make new friends

It is important to have someone to talk to about your concerns or anxieties. Who understands your situation more than a woman who is going through the same experience? If you are able to get out of bed, find a way to meet some of the other women on your floor. As I mentioned, I did this by organizing a pizza party. However, it may be as simple is introducing yourself to another mom while getting some water in the shared kitchen, connecting with your roommate, or making your way to the common lounge.

I met one of my friends while waiting for an ultrasound. We were both dressed in bathrobes (courtesy of an early appointment) so I made the right guess that she was in antenatal. Turns out she was in the room next to me. Since she was pregnant with triplets, she wasn't able to get out of her room much. Since I was able to walk short distances, I decided to go visit her. Through these visits we became good friends. Once her condition stabilized, she began pushing herself in a wheelchair to the common room and struck up friendships with some of the other women, particularly the moms carrying multiples. I'm always glad I made the effort to talk to her, and invited myself into her room, as she became a huge support for me after my son was born.

Someone needs to start the conversation — so why not you?

2. Visitors

As you enter the hospital, you might be thinking about how many people will come visit to help you pass the time. While visitors are great, a word of warning: They can also be exhausting. The main focus of your bed rest should be your baby and doing what is needed to keep baby healthy and growing; this often means resting.

I found that while I enjoyed visitors, there definitely was a limit to how many and how often. Since I was over an hour away from home, I had a lot fewer visitors than some women. However, even my small amount could wear me out — depending on the visitor and how long he or she stayed. I do know that for some of the moms, the amount of visitors did more harm than good, as it left them little time to rest.

So here are some basic rules for visitors:

- Ask friends/family to set up time in advance versus popping in.
- Limit the length of the visit before they arrive.
- Set up your own visiting hours (to ensure there is time for rest in between visits and medical tests).

When it comes to the question, "is there anything you'd like me to bring?" The answer should always be "yes"! Most people know it is basic etiquette to bring a gift when visiting someone in the hospital. If you aren't specific on the gift, you'll end up with a room full of candy, magazines, and flowers. Here are some practical items visitors can bring for you and to share with other moms on the floor:

- Home baked goodies such as muffins, cookies, and other treats
- Fresh fruit, fruit salads, or fruit bowls
- Fresh vegetable platters or cut up veggies
- Trail mix

- Crackers (as hospitals usually only have saltines)
- iTunes gift cards
- Netflix subscription
- Tablet carrying case
- Books
- Craft supplies

Stephanie's Story

Stephanie Keeping
Zero days on bed rest, but many days supporting a mom in hospital
Mother of one

While I had a relatively normal pregnancy with my son and didn't spend any time on bed rest, I did spend many days on the antenatal unit visiting my friend. So my story is more about providing advice to your family and friends, and is one I hope you will share with them. Sometimes it's better to hear from a stranger how they can help you.

One of the best things your support team can do is visit you — at home or in hospital. It's that simple. Just take the time to come see you. If distance is a challenge, they can jump on FaceTime or Skype. But they just need to visit.

Three times a week my son and I would drive 45 minutes to see our friend in the hospital. Yes, it was a trek, but I knew she needed the company. I'm from the east coast and live a couple of plane rides away from my family, so I know what's it's like to be separated from family during pregnancy.

None of my visits were "pop-ins," rather I made sure the time and day worked for my friend and didn't conflict with any of her tests or appointments. I also connected with her in advance to see if there was anything she wanted me to pick up at the grocery store as I had heard the horror stories of the hospital food. As she became friends with the moms on her floor, I started bringing treats she could share, such as cupcakes and fruit salad.

My son looked forward to these trips as they always involved either a visit to the children's indoor playground on the pediatric unit or a "swing ride" outside on one of the porch swings. In a way, these visits helped familiarize him with hospitals, letting him see they weren't a scary place but rather a place where people who were sick got the help they needed.

During our visits we also spent time in the common room with my friend and the other moms. They soon accepted me as an "honorary mom" and I was included in the group discussions. I was impressed with the strength of these women, who were all hours away from family and friends, but had somehow come together to support each other. Even though they were from different backgrounds, their shared experience made them friends.

I also heard the stories of siblings, parents, and friends who lived close to the hospital but never visited and the hurt their absence caused these women. Some of these friends lived a short drive away, but were too busy in their daily lives to make the trip to the hospital.

If you are able to visit, make the trip. Yes, it can be an inconvenience and challenging, but the time you can spend will mean the world to a mom who is confined to home or hospital-based bed rest. It will also strengthen your relationship, as she will know you truly care about her and her baby.

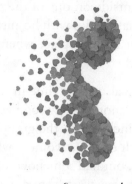

Chapter 24

Getting Ready for Baby

One of the upsides of being in a hospital is the potential access to a variety of healthcare professionals. The amount of access will depend on the size of your hospital.

While you are on bed rest, where possible, take advantage of these healthcare professionals. Ask if you can either have them come visit you in your room, or if you are on an antenatal unit, ask if an information session can be held in the common room for all of the moms.

The following sections discuss the individuals who may help you prepare for baby.

1. Lactation Nurse

If you're in a small hospital, a nurse from labor and delivery might be available for a one-on-one discussion. If you're on an antenatal unit, ask if a lactation session can be held for all the moms. Even if this isn't your first child, it is helpful to hear from a lactation nurse. The nurse will demonstrate proper latching, how to hand express, and discuss common breastfeeding challenges. Once again it is about sharing information and making personal connections. If you end up needing lactation support after baby is born, this connection will be important. The lactation nurse who held the information session on my unit ended up visiting me daily when I first had my son, helping me hand express milk for my husband to take to the NICU for his tube feedings.

2. Dietician

The rules about what to feed to baby at what age keep changing. While it's hard for parents to keep up with the changes, a dietician will know at what age babies should be exposed to peanuts, eggs, milk, and other potential allergens. Learning about the latest food introduction guidelines, and when to introduce solids, will help you better prepare for baby. Now is the time to access a dietician, as you will have little time once baby is born.

3. Physical Therapist

You've spent days or weeks lying in bed, and likely have more than a few aches and pains. Once baby is born you won't be jumping back on the treadmill, hitting the gym, or picking up where you left off. Now is the time to find out if there are any exercises or information the physical therapist can offer to help you on your road to recovery. Are there any exercises or activities you should avoid after baby is born? Are there any resources to get help or connect with other moms after you and baby are discharged? Some communities have exercise programs specific for new moms. Remember, these are aimed at low-risk moms. It may take your body a bit longer to get back in shape so don't push it too soon.

4. Public Health Unit

While in hospital, try to find out if your public health unit offers new baby visits. If so, it might be worth connecting with your local unit. Here's something I learned: Because I was in a large hospital outside of my community, my local health unit would have no way of knowing I'd had a baby as new baby files are only shared from the local hospital to the local health unit. Not out of town deliveries. While this makes sense, I hadn't thought about the fact I needed to reach out to my local health unit and register my son's birth. I was able to connect with the health unit from my hospital bed to set up a post-discharge visit.

5. Circumcision

Some hospitals offer circumcision for boys before they are discharged. If you are expecting a son and have made the decision to circumcise, you can make the necessary arrangements before your son is born, or at least find out the information on costs and risks and whether it is right for your son.

6. Self-Preparation

There is lots to be done when baby arrives. Why not do some of this work from your hospital bed?

Have you registered your baby for daycare? Now is a great time to research daycares in your community and start filling out the lengthy application forms.

Do you have other children? Once again, take this time to register them in any extracurricular or summer activities or research ways for them to spend their summer months. I was able to find a half-day summer camp near my home for my daughter to attend after I was discharged from the hospital. This would give her a fun activity in the morning, as well as give me time alone with my son.

Have you read about life with baby? Lots of times we read the pregnancy books but not the books about life with a baby. This is a great time to read books about sleeping, early development, and nutrition (for you and baby).

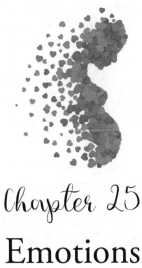

Chapter 25

Emotions

By now you are well aware that pregnancy and bed rest is an emotional time for mothers. Don't be scared or run away from these emotions as they are real and part of the journey. If there is any time in your life that people will completely understand you breaking down and crying for no reason, or experiencing a rollercoaster of mood swings, it is during pregnancy.

Add having your freedom taken away and being confined to bed rest in a hospital, and the emotional rollercoaster has a few additional hills and bends.

I've talked a lot about the importance of building your support network throughout this book. You know the saying — it takes a village to raise a child. For some of you, now is a good time to build or grow your village.

During your hospital stay it is great if some of you can make friends with other moms on your unit. If you don't, it's important to rely on your family and friends. You need the support now more than ever. Be honest with the people who make up your support system about what you're feeling and ask for help when you need it.

In my six weeks on antenatal I only saw the social worker once, for less than five minutes. She somehow forgot to visit me, and spent more time talking about her job than asking how I was doing. Even so, this was the only time during my hospital stay — in antenatal or NICU — that anyone asked me how I was doing emotionally. Looking back I find it odd, and disappointing, that no one ever checked in to see how I was coping mentally. All the conversations were about the baby and my physical health, but never about my mental health.

To be honest, I never talked about my emotions with my medical team. It didn't come up in their visits and I never brought it up. This doesn't mean I wasn't struggling. As I mentioned before there were lots of times where I would close my door and have a good, ugly cry. Even though nurses witnessed some of my breakdowns, they didn't take the time to ask if I was okay, as they were likely uncomfortable seeing the emotions.

There were also some traumatic events that happened on our floor and while the mother involved may have received support, the rest of us, who either witnessed or were aware of the event, did not. Instead we gathered in the common room, shared stories and had a good cry. I often wondered what support mothers receive who either haven't been able to make friends on the unit or are confined to their room due to their pregnancy complications.

There are many positive outcomes and pure miracles that happen in antenatal and the NICU, but there are also heartbreaking losses. Not every mother is able to bring her baby home. These losses have an impact on everyone, and sadly many hospitals do not have the resources to support those impacted by the loss.

I don't tell you this to scare you, but to make you aware that as a patient you need to ask for help rather than waiting for someone to come and check to see if you are okay. It is important to be your own advocate, and to advocate for other patients. If you feel uncomfortable doing this, talk to your partner or a friend and have him or her speak to your medical team on your behalf. Or make friends with a nurse who you can confide in and have the candid conversations.

Looking back, I wish the medical team on our antenatal unit had provided us moms with support when one of our moms delivered an angel baby (a baby who dies in utero, shortly after delivery or a stillborn). We had become friends and knew the ups and downs of her pregnancy. We also all shared in her loss. In the absence of support, we became our own support group, and did our best to help the mom. Mothers, who had also suffered late term losses, were able to provide her additional support, not only emotionally, but also the realities of burying her angel baby.

After my son was born, I learned the importance of not only having a support system but also leaning on others during difficult times. Like the experience I talked about in home-based bed rest, I had my breaking point moment when my son was in NICU.

A friend had come to visit me, and my son's nurse told her I wasn't at the hospital, despite the fact I was sitting at my son's bedside. She had mixed me up with another mom (even though she only had three patients) so she turned away my visitor. Being more than an hour away from home, I had few visitors during my two months in hospital, and each one was a valued distraction.

Hearing my visitor had been turned away and having no way of contacting her, as I didn't have a cell phone, was my breaking point. My weeks in the hospital and all I had gone through finally caught up with me. I broke down and cried. This was the ugly crying I talked about. It wasn't pretty. My son's nurse felt horrible and I didn't care.

In a blur I walked down to antenatal into the room of a mom friend, my former hospital room neighbor. At first the nurses tried to tell me to leave, as my friend was in early stages of labor and having her own rough day. Being a crying mess they let me stay. I sat beside my friend bawling my eyes out while she was breathing through labor pains with two nurses hovering over her.

For the hour I spent at her bedside we never spoke. I kept crying and she kept breathing. Just being there with someone who knew what I was going through, even without us talking, meant so much. When I was done my meltdown I stood up, gave her a huge hug and went back to the NICU to see my beautiful son.

The following day when I went back to see her, her labor had slowed down and I had resumed my NICU routine (pumping, feeding, cuddling, and resting). We had a good talk about my visit, and all the stresses of having a baby in NICU. A few days later she delivered her two daughters, who joined us for a short stay in the NICU.

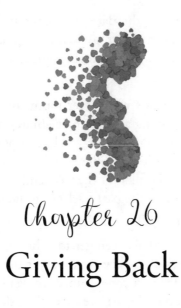

Chapter 26

Giving Back

Although it may seem that you'll never get out of the hospital and resume your normal life, at some point you will have your baby or babies, and leave the confines of your hospital room for your own comfortable bed at home. While your main focus for the next few months will be caring for your new baby and reconnecting with your children, once you have settled into a routine you may be wondering how you can give back to the hospital, community, and/or support system that helped you during your journey.

Some moms throw thank-you parties for their support system; an open house/meet the baby/thank you for your help party. This is a great way to say a big joint thank you to everyone who helped look after your children, cooked meals, visited you in the hospital, or played a role in supporting you and your family during your bed rest.

If this is something that interests you, now is a great time to start planning for this party, while you have some time lying in bed. Who would you invite? Is there a theme? What food would you serve? Do you want your guests to sign a book, leave a video message, or sign a picture frame with a welcoming message to your baby? Where would you hold this party? Can you make and address the invitations now, holding off on filling in the date and time? Planning a thank you party can be a great distraction as well as a good way to graciously accept the help you need now, knowing you can thank everyone later for their support.

If you've made friends with other moms on your unit, you can spend some time planning a party to celebrate the baby's first birthday. One of the moms on my unit owned a campground on the shores of Lake Huron in Ontario. She offered to host the party, putting each family up in a camping trailer for the weekend. We spent hours in the common room planning the party, selecting the date, and looking at pictures of her campground.

We also planned a Halloween get-together so we could reconnect and see all the babies after they were out of the NICU (our babies were born in late May and June). Since we were from various communities, up to four hours apart, we spent time determining the most central location. We finally found a community hall to rent near one of the mom's homes, where we would have room for our older kids to run around and a warm spot for us to meet with our babies.

I have known some moms who have volunteered at Ronald McDonald House, cooking a meal for families staying there, as they too spent many a nights at this great facility.

For those of you not familiar with Ronald McDonald House, it is a home away from home for families with babies or children getting care in the hospital. These low-cost houses are often located near large, regional hospitals with pediatric units or children's hospitals.

I knew very little about Ronald McDonald House until my son was admitted into NICU and the nurse told my husband he needed to book us a room to stay until my son was discharged. In our case, the house was located next to the hospital's parking lot, only a few steps from the front entrance to the Children's Hospital.

Parents looking to stay need a referral from the medical staff. In many cases this is a simple phone call from the unit nurse to staff at the house confirming you have a child in care and the anticipated length of stay. For $10 a night (cost may vary at different locations) we had a hotel-like room to sleep, all of our food was provided, parking was included, and there were common areas for friends and family to visit. This included a playroom for when our daughter came to see us. The close location to the hospital meant I could go to the house for homemade meals, without being far away from my son. It also saved me from having to spend a fortune eating in the hospital cafeteria.

During my stay at Ronald McDonald House, I was served dinner one night by a woman I had previously worked with almost a decade earlier. She told me when her twin daughters were born; she spent a few weeks at Ronald McDonald House while they were in the NICU. She always remembered the support she and her husband received during their difficult time, and promised to give back when she was able.

Once her daughters got older, she and a group of friends began making monthly meals at Ronald McDonald House. Her daughters, who were now in their twenties, joined her. Her one daughter is now a nurse in the pediatric unit at the hospital. It has all come full circle.

I was approached by my OB during my hospital stay to sit as a patient advocate on the perinatal council. This is a decision-making committee made up of doctors, nurses, and midwives from labor and delivery, the antenatal and maternity units, as well as the NICU. While the committee had the necessary medical staff, they were looking for a member who could bring the patient's perspective. My OB, who knew I wasn't shy on sharing my opinions and advocating for patients, asked me to join the committee once I was discharged and when I felt I had the time to commit.

When my son was three months old, I attended my first committee meeting. I spent the next three years attending quarterly meetings, making the one-hour drive to the hospital. I truly enjoyed my time on this to not only give back to the hospital that had taken such great care of my son and I, but also to help other parents in their journey. My weeks in the hospital had provided a unique insight to hospital life and a perspective that is often not seen by the medical staff.

My work on this committee also opened up opportunities to provide feedback to the Ministry of Health in relation to maternal care. I helped develop a post-discharge for new moms to provide feedback on their time in hospital, aimed at improving care.

The time I spent on the committee also improved my confidence as a patient advocate and gave me insider knowledge of the medical system. This has helped me in continuing to advocate for my son, who has some challenges.

While I sadly had to resign from this committee when I moved across the country, I was grateful for the time and ability to give back to the hospital that had given me the most precious gift of all — my son.

I admit the idea of giving back may be overwhelming right now as you are doing your best to incubate and wait until as close to your due date as possible before delivering. I'm not asking you to make any firm commitments, but rather think about how you can say thank you to your support system, continue the connections you've made, or help other moms in the future.

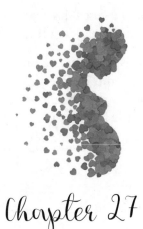

Chapter 27

Final Thoughts

I hope this book, if nothing else, has helped you pass a few hours of your bed rest. I also hope it has made you take some time to not only reflect on your situation, but also make some plans for getting help and preparing for baby. Most of all, I hope you realize you are not alone in your journey.

Right now, there are women all over the world in your same situation. Many have the same fears, anxieties, and excitement. Many are feeling alone, as if they are the only person struggling with these emotions.

Women are amazing communicators and healers. Unfortunately we are also good at putting on a brave face and not asking for help when we need it most.

Pregnancy is an incredible way to bond with coworkers, friends, family, and your community. You will be surprised at how many people will do just about anything to help a pregnant woman. All you need to do is reach out, share your experience with them, and let them know the specific help you need.

Whether you're on bed rest for a few days or a few months, the best you can do is take it one day at a time.

Remember the words a wise nurse once told me: Every day you give your baby in your womb is a blessing. Don't look at how many days you have left until you reach full term, but how many days of love you have given your baby. Take your bed rest day by day.

I wish you nothing but love and support as you give your baby one more day of rest and growing time.

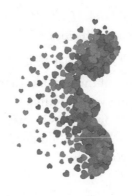

Appendix

Recommended Reading

The Oh She Glows Cookbook by Angela Liddon (Penguin Canada, 2014). Even if you aren't a vegan, you will love this *New York Times* bestselling cookbook. It features more than 100 plant-based recipes that are easy to make and are hits for the whole family. While you likely aren't cooking now, it's a good book to help you understand the importance of a whole food diet (non-processed meals made with real ingredients) and flag some recipes for when you are on your feet again. She has two cookbooks, so get out your sticky notes and begin flagging your favorite recipes.

Chocolate-Covered Katie by Katie Higgins (Grand Central Life & Style, 2015). This is my go-to baking cookbook. The writer has a sweet tooth, with chocolate being her favorite sweet. The recipes are healthy takes on desserts, with classics such as black bean brownies, chickpea blondies, and yummy butterfingers. Before you roll your eyes at the ingredients, trust me, the recipes are tasty and kid-approved. When my kids see me bringing out this cookbook they put on their aprons and are excited to see what treats we will bake. Amazon ranked her first cookbook as one of the Top 20 Cookbooks of 2015. Her second cookbook, *Hello Breakfast*, is filled with family friendly and yummy breakfast recipes.

You: Raising Your Child by Michael F. Roizen and Mehmet C. Oz (Scriber, 2010). This is one of those books that will become a staple in your house as you're raising your children. I first borrowed this book from the library, but then bought it as it was such a handy resource. It has some great information about child development, healthy eating, and exercises to do with your kids.

Websites

Birth Plan Templates

Birth Plan Template

    www.womenshealthcaretopics.com/BirthPlanTemplate.html

MyBirthPlan.com Template

    www.mybirthplan.com/wp-content/uploads/2016/05/ Birth-Plan.pdf

Visual Birth Plan Template

    www.mamanatural.com/visual-birth-plan

Baby Resources

Baby Center

    www.babycenter.com

Today's Parent

    www.todaysparent.com

Ronald McDonald House

United States

    www.rmhc.org

Canada

    http://rmhbc.ca

Mom's Mental Health

BC Children's Hospital: This Canadian site covers the spectrum of pre-pregnancy, pregnancy, postpartum, pregnancy loss, infertility, and PMS with many great resources for women and their families.

https://reproductivementalhealth.ca

Royal College of Psychiatrists: This site out of the United Kingdom is aimed at improving the lives of people with mental illness.

www.rcpsych.ac.uk/healthadvice/problemsdisorders/mental healthinpregnancy.aspx

Beyond Blue: This Australian website provides online resources and support for pregnancy, new parents as well as building healthy families.

https://healthyfamilies.beyondblue.org.au/pregnancy-and-new-parents/maternal-mental-health-and-wellbeing